You Oughta Know

Acknowledging, Recognizing, and Responding to the Steps in the Journey Through Dementias and Alzheimer's Disease

By

Sandra Ross

© 2014

Table of Contents

Forward

This book takes a comprehensive look at each of the steps in the journey through dementias and Alzheimer's Disease. I've seen, in my own experience (I went, side-by-side, through the journey of vascular dementia, Lewy Body dementia, and Alzheimer's Disease with my mom all the way through the end of her life) and in supporting, educating, and counseling others who are on the journey, that there is a basic lack of comprehension about the big picture of how these neurological diseases progress.

My purpose here is to lay that big picture out in concrete and discrete steps that follow this pattern for each step:

1. What is happening
2. What it looks like
3. How to address it

I cannot emphasis enough that a timely intervention that consists of geriatric psychiatric hospitalization where an accurate diagnosis can be made and a medication regimen to address cognition, psychological issues, moods, behaviors, and psychosis started (it will be tweaked along the way), along with our love and advocacy, can minimize and stabilize a lot of these and increase the quality of our loved one's lives.

This should be done sooner rather than later. It won't cure dementias and Alzheimer's Disease. There is no cure for these neurological diseases. They are always fatal.

However, the proper medication regimen can increase the quality of life for our loved ones in a way that gives them an opportunity to live life as fully as they're able, to enjoy it as much as they're able, and to enjoy their relationships with those they love, including us. The goal is to stabilize, not marginalize or invisibalize (being almost comatose is not quality of life), so it's our job to find the right medical care team to make this happen for our loved ones.

Waiting only hurts them and endangers their lives. And it could end their lives prematurely. None of us want that. So, I urge you to get psychiatric help and medication on board as soon as possible!

The tone of this book is conversational. As I'm writing it, I'm imagining each of you reading it sitting beside me, across from me, as we share a cup of coffee or a glass of tea, talking as friends.

Because we are, even though you and I have never met in person.

I know intimately the struggles you're dealing with now, as well as the struggles your loved ones are dealing with. I know the sense of helplessness you and they wrestle with. I know the deep, deep desire to fix it, to make it better, to wave a magic wand and make it disappear.

I know the moments of great sorrow and the moments of great joy you and your loved ones share. I also know the great love you have for each other.

And I know the battles you are going to face after this journey is over. It changes you forever. But the lessons you'll learn are the ones that you will share with others, as I'm sharing mine with you. To not pay them forward is to waste the pain.

If you have not yet read my practical and loving caregiving book, *Going Gentle Into That Good Night* (available on Amazon in paperback and Kindle versions, please be sure to purchase that as well). For regular updates and new information on dementias and Alzheimer's Disease, please subscribe to my blog at http://goinggentleintothatgoodnight.com.

As always, if you have any questions that I can help you with or you just need someone to listen, please email me at goinggentleintothatgoodnight@gmail.com.

Love and prayers for each of you,

Sandra

Chapter 1: "I Don't Remember, I Don't Recall"

The first step of the journey into dementias and Alzheimer's Disease (Alzheimer's Disease is a form of dementia, but all dementias are not Alzheimer's Disease) is usually mild cognitive impairment, characterized by short-term memory loss.

Mild cognitive impairment does not always mean that dementia and Alzheimer's Disease is right around the corner. Part of what causes mild cognitive impairment, especially in older people, is natural aging of the brain and their slowing down in a world that is speeding up around them, making it almost impossible for them to keep up.

When my mom's mild cognitive impairment first began to be sporadically apparent, because I have been in information technology for my entire career, I used to tell her that she needed her hard drive (brain) cleaned up and optimized and she needed a memory (because hers was full) upgrade.

For someone with non-dementia and non-Alzheimer's Disease, that is a snapshot of what mild cognitive impairment is.

Because it affects short-term memory, mild cognitive impairment affects the recent past and the present.

What does this look like in practical terms?

1. Repeating things in conversations, stories, and writing

    This manifests itself in telling the same things over and over, and with each retelling, it's as though it's the first time telling it. It is very similar to the effect of a scratch in an old vinyl record, where that point in the track gets replayed over and over until someone goes over and physically lifts the needle up and moves it beyond the scratch. However, with our loved ones, it's rarely that easy or that simple.

2. Frequently losing and misplacing things

We all, from time to time, pick things up, get derailed in going from point A to point B, laying the things down somewhere in between, and then having no idea where we put them when we finally get to point B. However, with mild cognitive impairment, this becomes normal.

For the longest time with my mom, I thought this was just a side effect of her jumping from one thing to another (something I never was acutely aware of about Mom until after my dad died, and I realized he'd been the focuser, the organizer, and the goal/task manager in their relationship). I chalked it up to her hearing loss and the way she learned to hide/cope with it until she got hearing aids in her mid-20's by anticipating what she needed to do or say next and moving to that before she got behind.

But then it began happening a lot. With everything.

I think I really became conscious that Mom had mild cognitive impairment when she was still living independently in her retirement community. I had stopped by one day after to work to spend the evening with her as I did every day and she was in a panic when I walked in.

I asked what was wrong and she said she couldn't find her wallet with her credit cards. I asked her when the last time was that she'd seen it and she told me it was in her purse earlier that day.

I literally spent two hours combing every inch of her living space looking for it and I couldn't find it either. I then got on the phone and canceled all the cards and decided to keep just one credit card (the one she'd had the longest) and her debit card and put myself as the secondary contact on them to simplify things if this happened again.

Fortunately, no one had used any of the missing cards, and to do this day, I have no idea what happened to the wallet.

3. Forgetting recent conversations

   "I just told you that _____." Within a recent timeframe, finding ourselves saying this a lot is probably a good indicator that mild cognitive impairment is in play. The other part of this is from our loved ones: "You never told me that."

This is an argument we will not win. All the logic, all the attempts to stimulate remembering will not work.

It took me a while not to get upset and it took even longer for me to not question my own sanity and memory ("Did I really say that or did I just think I said that?") when Mom and I would have impasses over recent conversations.

It took a while, but I realized it wasn't her fault and she wasn't trying to argue with me just to be arguing with me, but this one was, for me, early on one of the most maddening aspects of Mom's mild cognitive impairment.

4. Frequently losing train of thought in conversations

For those of us that think a lot and talk a little (I'm one of them), there are occasions where, as we're trying to give a cogent and concise explanation of our thought processes, we tend to lose our train of thought in conversations. I have analyzed this and why it happens to me and I have realized that it occurs because of the constant back and forth between retrieving thoughts, organizing them, and then processing the organized thoughts into speech. It's a complex, tedious, and time-consuming process and is fraught with the propensity to forget where you are in the process.

Ironically, I suspect that's the same kind problem that occurs with our loved ones who have mild cognitive impairment with a few more wrinkles thrown in. Because mild cognitive impairment is, at the least, an aging brain and more likely, a sign of neurological damage related to dementias and Alzheimer's Disease, not only is the actual process of retrieval, organization, and speech harder, but there are actual gaps in the neurological network where either information is missing or the route to get to it (as in vascular dementia, where the brain will try to find an alternate pathway to stored information, but it's often long and circuitous) is long and trying.

This is where we often find half-spoken sentences trail off into nothing, the wrong words used to describe people, places, and things, and a level of frustration, especially if impatience is encountered (we have to do our best not to finish the sentences, but instead listen attentively and just wait for them as long as it takes) that can lead to our loved ones giving up on communication at all.

5. Inability to keep up with the thread of conversations

The most obvious sign of this is when someone with mild cognitive impairment suddenly injects something into a conversation that makes absolutely no sense. What we find is that keeping up with the thread of conversations among a group of people is most difficult.

With time and patience, one-on-one conversations can continue quite effectively. But with mild cognitive impairment, essentially what's happening in the brain with multiple people and conversations (or even TV or music in the background) is information overload with no place to go.

Since short-term memory is affected, little snippets of incomplete information are assaulting the brains of our loved ones, making confusion and frustration worse. People with mild cognitive impairment will tend to get extremely quiet and they will mentally either shut down or go to a place in their own thinking that is safe and comfortable. When things quieten down, they will speak, but the speech contains a piece of information from that safe and comfortable place, which will likely not have anything to do with the current conversations.

It's our job to be aware of when this is happening. We need to do our best to ensure a quieter environment for our loved ones (I often would walk with Mom into another room and we'd sit down together for a while) and then engage our loved ones in one-on-one conversations. By doing this we can ease a lot of anxiety and we can also keep them in the present longer. And most of all, by doing this, we say "I love you and I care about you."

6. Being consistently overwhelmed when faced with decision-making, making plans to complete an action, or processing instructions into action

This part of mild cognitive impairment can be hard to discern in some of our loved ones, especially if this is an area where they've had difficulties all their lives, especially when it comes to decision-making and planning. Some people, by temperament or personality, just ever don't do this easily or well.

However, the one facet that usually brings this area to a head is that of processing instructions into action.

Mom had always been decisive, but she took her time and got a lot of input from others before making decisions. It always seemed to be a bit of a paralytic process for her, even when she was younger and on top of things.

Again, my dad helped guide the process most of the time, so the only times I ever saw the paralytic side of this was when Dad was gone (he spent the better part of a year when we were little working as a field veterinarian handling large animal disease control in another part of the state we lived in, so he was gone for long stretches of time, leaving Mom to handle the decision-making on her own in his absence).

After Dad's death, I stepped in to help Mom out in this area. With enough input and time, she'd reach a decision and all seemed to be normal for long stretches of time.

Mom handled planning adequately, but it was never her strong suite. But, still, it was hard for me to see any discernable problems for quite a while.

But processing instructions into action was something Mom had always been very good at. As a microbiologist and a medical technologist, one of the real strengths she brought to her studies and her profession was the ability to retain, comprehend, and execute existing and new instructions rapidly, easily, and accurately.

And it was Mom's loss of ability to do this with any kind of ease, no matter how many times or ways I explained something, how easily and logically I spelled them out step-by-step, that I really became aware of the problem. Mom began to not be able to do this at all with new information. Mom could still do it somewhat well with things she already knew how to do, but even there I could see a difference.

The foremost example of this was when we set up an online banking account for Mom. We did this so that I could help her keep track of bills, checks, and make sure her bank accounts were up-to-date.

I painstakingly wrote detailed, easy-to-follow (I broke every action out into a numbered step instead of combining the obvious ones), step-by-step instructions for Mom to log in to her account. I set up a bookmark in her browser to take her right where she needed to be to log in. I sat down with Mom every day for a week, having her do the computer work, walking her slowly through each step in the instructions.

And I thought Mom had it. Until I went over on a Sunday morning and Mom was in tears because none of it made sense to her and she couldn't remember how to do it. I began to try to walk Mom through it again, paying attention this time to her and how she was reacting and I realized then that she couldn't do it. I knew it wasn't sticking and I realized in that instant how frustrating it was for Mom.

From then on, Mom sat beside me while I logged in and we went through the checkbook together a few times until that got frustrating for her, and then I just had Mom sit beside me once a week while I took the checkbook and went through her online account to make sure everything matched.

7. Losing track of time

Older folks, in general, seem to be less concerned with time passing than we younger folks are. We live in a world where everything runs on time. We have a ton of technology that helps us keep track of time, reminds us of time, and causes us anxiety if we're out of time.

However, with mild cognitive impairment, not only is there less concern with time, but there is an actual loss of time.

Part of the problem is with the actual telling of time. Most of the cognitive tests include drawing a clock from memory, putting the numbers on it properly, and drawing the long hand and short hand to match a specific time. When mild cognitive impairment is present, this becomes extremely difficult to do. Here are a couple of examples of this exercise where mild cognitive impairment is present:

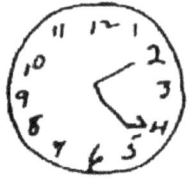 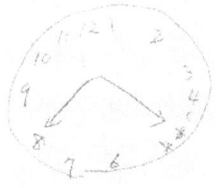

I remember Mom showing me – a rare feat in itself in those days of secretiveness about her doctors'

appointments - the test that her doctor had given her that included this exercise (her number placement was more askew and messier than the diagram on the right, and she had the long and short hands reversed, but in the general area where the hands should have been) and I was shocked. She was having trouble with time using an analog clock.

Looking back, I'm sure she had to depend on light to know whether it was daytime or nighttime and the rest was just a best guess.

Interestingly, I don't remember Mom ever being late for anything we were doing together, but I always checked in with her beforehand too. There were times, however, when she just took off without me, so I have to wonder if this was part of the problem.

In the mild cognitive impairment stage, the easiest solution in the short-term is to buy a 24-hour digital clock with the date and time and have it nearby so our loved ones can always look at it and know the exact time and date and time of day.

I have wondered, as a side note, what kind of test, if time goes on long enough, will have to be developed for the Millennial generation which has had nothing but digital time all their lives. My guess is that a lot of them wouldn't be to draw an analog clock with no cognitive impairment.

8. Difficulty learning new things

   This goes hand-in-hand with #6, where I discuss it.

9. Difficulty remembering new information

   This also goes hand-in-hand with #6.

10. Forgetting to do daily, repetitive tasks like taking medication, paying bills, or keeping appointments

    Skipping medication or forgetting to get prescriptions filled is usually one of the first signs in this area of mild cognitive impairment. So are unpaid bills and missed appointments.

    With Mom, I was already helping keep up with bills and appointments, when medication began to be a problem, even though I was involved to a degree with that as well.

    After Mom's hospitalizations in 2008, I bought a dry erase board and put it on the refrigerator and kept a current list, written large enough for her to easily see, of her morning and nighttime medications. I would put the name and the dose, so we both knew what she was taking, when she was taking it, and how much (I needed this every time we went to the hospital, so it was helpful for me too) she was taking.

That worked well for about a year, but then Mom asked me if I would help her put keep up with the daily medications. I bought a weekly medication holder with AM and PM sections and each Sunday, I'd fill it for the week.

Not long after I started doing this for Mom, I noticed as I was doing a Sunday refill that there were days from the previous week where she had not taking her medication in the morning or in the evening. It was erratic, but it concerned me because everything Mom was on was something she needed to take every day.

The way I handled this until Mom decided she was going to stop all the medication "with her doctor's approval" (things were so combustible then that I did everything in my power to keep things from blowing up spontaneously; I simply knew this was not something I could change her mind on and, even though I knew she could die as a result, it would have been a fiercely hellacious and losing battle and she would have pushed me even further away) was to literally check in the morning and evening of each day to make sure that Mom had taken her medication. If she hadn't, then I'd get a glass of water and hand it to her to take it while I was there.

11. Frequently forgetting what they're doing, such as cooking and forgetting the stove is on and burning the

food or setting off smoke alarms, or leaving the car running with the keys locked inside while they're running errands

For our loved ones with mild cognitive impairment, it's easy to get sidetracked and forget about an earlier task, such as cooking, or to forget to turn the ignition off before getting out of the car. Admittedly, I have done both of these at least once in my life, but it's not a frequent occurrence and I realized as soon as I'd done it (as in the case of locking my keys in the car with the ignition running – I actually had a legitimate reason to leave the car running because I was trying to see if the problem with my phone not charging was the battery or the charger).

However when this kind of forgetfulness occurs frequently, then it is likely evidence of mild cognitive impairment. This one can be a difficult one to manage without affecting our loved ones' independence, but offering to share tasks such as cooking and running errands gives us the ability to oversee and prevent any danger while helping out, and it still gives our loved ones the independence to do as many of their daily activities as they're able.

It's important, though, not to take over and not to scold. "Why don't we_____?" works very effectively and it lets our loved ones know that they and we are a team.

12. Having trouble navigating in familiar surroundings

Driving is where this is most obvious and happens frequently. With mild cognitive impairment, our loved ones can often forget how to get from one point to another on a very familiar route and will drive around until they are totally lost.

The other activity this can be a problem with is walking, especially if our loved ones are used to taking walks every day.

Again, it's imperative not to scold. However it may be time to, in the case of driving, ask the family physician to state to our loved ones that for safety reasons it's time to give up driving (we need to make sure we're available to get our loved ones out and about as much and often as they want or need to be).

With walking, it is simply a matter of walking with them to ensure they are safe (and everybody can use more exercise!).

13. Exercising less impulse control

One of the first signs of mild cognitive impairment is the evidence of "filters" in the brain being turned off.

We all think and feel things that we never verbalize or act on. In fact, there are many things that we reject before they even take root in our thinking. Those are the "filters" a healthy brain has that are developed by nurture and environment all our lives.

Small children don't start out with these "filters," which is why they hear things like "you shouldn't say that" or "you shouldn't act like that" with explanations as to why while they're growing up.

Because of the neurological damage of mild cognitive impairment, these lifetime "filters" either get damaged, destroyed, or are simply impossible neurologically to get to. Therefore, it's not uncommon for our loved ones to start cursing a blue streak, crying spontaneously and hysterically, laughing inappropriately, verbalizing everything they're thinking and feeling with brutal honesty, and throwing temper tantrums.

I know from first-hand experience this is one of the most shocking things to deal with. Mom's signs were crying, verbalizing everything she was thinking and feeling, and throwing temper tantrums when she was in this stage and as the disease progressed until we were able to get medication to help with cognition. I never got over the shock, even when I realized this was our present reality at the time. I still always surprised me.

I've talked with friends whose mothers had dementias and Alzheimer's Disease and I heard similar stories.

One friend's mother (who was also one of Mom's best friends), a retired administrator, was the absolute epitome of self-control and grace until Alzheimer's Disease took over.

Then it was not uncommon for her to loudly label people, in public, as "bitches," "sons of bitches," and "bastards."

Another friend's mother, a registered nurse, had been a staunch supporter of civil rights in a southern city at the height of the racial conflict that followed the implementation of the 1964 Civil Rights Act, choosing to be one of the few white employees of one of the city's major hospitals to go on strike with the hospital's African-American employees, who were demanding better pay and better working conditions.

Therefore, it was quite shocking and embarrassing, when her mother, after dementia had set in, called one of the African-American in-home aides the "N" word to her face.

This is a tough one, but getting visibly upset and jumping all over our loved ones will make it worse. The reality is they don't know what they're doing and the moment goes as quickly as it comes and there is no memory of it. So, the easiest way to handle this with others is to apologize, explain what's going on, and let them know that our loved ones don't mean what they're saying.

One of the other aspects of poor impulse control can be sexual in nature (Mom didn't exhibit any of this, but it's not uncommon): taking clothes off in public and being sexually inappropriate in remarks and actions toward others.

Most of the research suggests that there are some underlying non-sexual reasons for this kind of poor impulse control. It is important to figure out what those are and make sure that those are addressed immediately. Some pharmacological research has shown that serotonin uptake inhibitors work effectively on these behaviors if they persist.

It is, above all else, imperative to consider the welfare of others if this is part of our loved ones' poor impulse control, and keep others safe at all times. That should be the number one concern in every situation.

14. Showing poor judgment

Showing poor judgment can manifest itself in numerous ways. With mild cognitive impairment, our loved ones are still able to function, in most situations, fairly independently, but because judgment is affected by neurological changes, they can make poor decisions in critical situations.

This makes them particularly vulnerable to being taken advantage of. The earliest evidence I have on my Mom's mild cognitive impairment (although at the time I didn't realize that was what was going on) was a situation in which she let three people she didn't know – they had knocked on the door and asked to use the phone - into the house we were sharing while I was at work. The three people immediately split up once they were inside and Mom couldn't keep an eye on them all. One person used the phone and then they left.

As soon as they were gone, Mom looked in her purse, which was in a different room than the phone, and her wallet was gone. Fortunately, I got home from work a short time later, but Mom was already in a panic about everything.

The most surprising thing to me initially was that my normally-very-careful-and-quite-suspicious-of-strangers Mom had let three strangers in the house to begin with. It was totally out of her character to do that. I knew that but I hadn't seen any other evidence of poor judgment on her part, so, at the time, I attributed it to Mom being from the old South where you helped people out whenever you could (in fact, that's why she told me she let them in).

We got on the phone immediately – I put the speaker on so Mom could hear and also so she could give the credit card companies permission to speak to me - and started canceling all the credit cards. Each card had been used within the hour at various local stores until a total of about $5000 had been charged. The last credit company I called showed that the charge on that card had been made just a minute or so earlier, so they got the police involved and the three people were arrested in that store.

Mom, of course, was not liable for any of the charges, but it concerned me and it scared her.

Even though I didn't realize what was going on, I handled it the way we should handle poor judgment. I let her talk through everything several times until she got calmed down. I reassured her over and over that everything was fine and the situation was all right.

I also took what she told me about just trying to help and approached it from the angle that the world was a different place than when she grew up and it wasn't safe to let people in our homes that we didn't know, no matter what the reason they gave.

Then I told her that she needed to look and see who was outside before she opened the door. If she didn't recognize them, then she needed to call 911. That way if they really did need help, then they'd have someone there right away who could help them.

I kept my voice calm and gentle and I held her hand while we were talking so she knew that I wasn't lecturing her and I wasn't giving her a hard time. I also didn't want her to beat up on herself.

At this point, gentleness combined with logic can often help somewhat with poor judgment in mild cognitive impairment. As dementias and Alzheimer's Disease progress, it will be less effective, but we cross those bridges when we get to them.

So what's the take away of how we address the issues that arise in mild cognitive impairment? This is where we can make this step better or worse.

The first response we have to this will likely be impatience, irritation and frustration.

That's because accepting a change like this in someone we love is very difficult. It brings mortality from a nether distance right into our faces. It signifies loss. It signifies a change in the relationship. And none of us are ever really ready for that.

As I've worked with others in a support, educational and counseling role, one of the most common statements about mild cognitive impairment is the suggestion that the person suffering with it is "doing it on purpose."

Let me tell you definitively that they are not doing this on purpose. There are no evil mechinations at work, no conscious manipulations, and no malevolent intents. This is simply what mild neurological degeneration looks like in action.

Because of our impatience, frustration, and irritation, the knee-jerk reaction will be to completely take over and take all independence away from our loved ones suffering with mild cognitive impairment.

This will be the worst possible thing we could do!

Imagine that today somebody came into your life and took every bit of independence, control, and freedom away from you. How would that affect you?

Now apply that to our loved ones with mild cognitive impairment. Every step of this journey requires walking in the other person's shoes. Without it, we cannot successfully and lovingly walk the journey with our loved ones.

Therefore, our best course of action for dealing effectively and kindly and gently with mild cognitive impairment is to make things easier for our loved ones suffering with it to be independent. This requires time and investment and diligence.

It's up to us to take the time, make the investment and be diligent. The longer our loved ones can stay independent and functioning, the better it will be for them.

As I've shown in many of the areas listed above, one of the best things that we can do is to team up with our loved ones in areas where they need help. It's imperative that we let them do as much as they can on their own, with us in more of an overseeing and coaching role, rather than taking over and not letting them do anything.

I've seen this happen and the decline is faster and worse once our loved ones have nothing to do and all control and independence is taken away from them.

Again, the most important thing I think we can all remember to do is to put ourselves in their shoes and imagine what it would be like for us to have absolutely no control over or independence in our lives. It takes longer. It takes patience. But it is so worth it!

Chapter 2: "There's Someone in My Head, But It's Not Me"

In this stage of dementias and Alzheimer's Disease, where mild cognitive impairment is more obvious, but the extensive neurological damage characterized by the later steps in these diseases has not yet occurred, most of the time our loved ones will function fairly normally and will be lucid.

However, they have an, sometimes quite acute, awareness of their own mental slippage and that something is not quite right. In other words, they are aware they can't remember things, they are losing things, they are having trouble following directions, and they can't seem to hold on to new information for any length of time.

After my dad died, Mom filled the huge void his death left by staying busy. Mom made meticulous notes in notebooks of things she needed to do, what she was researching, what she was learning in the continuing education classes she was taking at the local university, all the things she and I talked about in our daily conversations – her questions and my answers – and her private thoughts.

As I went through those notebooks before writing *Fields of Gold: A Love Story* (our family memoir) just after her death, I was surprised to come across a private thought she'd written in 2001, noting that she was having trouble keeping up with days of the week and wondering if she had Alzheimer's Disease.

Though it would be several more years before the signs of mild cognitive impairment were obvious and she was more acutely aware that something pervasively was wrong with her brain, that early wondering made me realize she was very self-aware of her own mental status and changes.

As these neurological diseases progress, our loved ones know something is changing or wrong, but they don't know what to do about it or how to fix it. This will often result in one of the following reactions from them:

1. Pretending it doesn't exist

    There is default wiring in human beings that tells them if they don't admit something, then it's not real. The presence of the signs of dementias and Alzheimer's Disease is no different in most people. This will manifest itself in a couple of ways.

    One manifestation is refusal to accept any help followed by the assertion that nothing is wrong and people are just trying to get their money, find something wrong, or take over and spend their money. There is a stubborn, insistent quest for complete independence that goes hand in hand with this refusal and rebuffing of genuine help.

    The other manifestation is that when something goes wrong, it's always someone else's fault. Because for our loved ones with these diseases accepting that they have the problem makes it real, the only option they have to explain and justify incidents and accidents is to blame others.

No one is immune from the blame. Generally, though, we, the people who are closest to them and who try to help the most, get the lion's share. Everything gets turned back on us and we become the bad guys.

This is, admittedly, a difficult thing for us to handle. We know our loved ones need help, but when we try to suggest or offer it, we get rebuffed unceremoniously or our loved ones turn the tables on us and we are the sole objects of their blame for just about everything that has happened and is happening in their lives. The accusations can get brutal as motives, designs, and intrigues are attributed to us that simply are not true and there is no logical way to reason or discuss this with our loved ones.

Remember that this is not personal and our loved ones aren't doing this on purpose. It is the effect of neurological damage that they have absolutely no control over.

Therefore, the first most prudent thing to do is to not engage. This requires a lot of self-control for us humans, because no one likes to be blamed for something that's not true and our gut reaction is to vigorously object and defend ourselves.

With our loved ones suffering from dementias and Alzheimer's Disease, all this will do is escalate the situation. It is our paramount duty not to do that. Escalation will only make it all worse.

The second most prudent thing to do is to calmly and quietly reassure our loved ones that we love them unconditionally (this will likely generate another round of blame and hostility, but it's imperative to never leave a conversation or a room with our loved ones without letting them know they are loved unconditionally) and take a physical break from the blame. It doesn't have to be a long break, but enough to give the mental state a chance to change.

Why remind our loved ones we love them unconditionally at a time when they are most unlovable? Well, for one, that's what they did with us when we were kids. But the more important reason is because none of us ever know what the last conversation we will have with someone will consist of. Not getting a chance for the last thing our loved ones hear and we say is "I love you unconditionally" is, in my opinion, the worst thing either of us would have to deal with.

2. Fear and/or stress

Fear and/or stress are often marked by panic and anxiety, and it is no different with our loved ones who are aware there is something neurologically wrong.

Panic and anxiety in healthy people causes more stress – which affects mental functioning – so when it happens to our loved ones with dementias and Alzheimer's Disease, you may see sudden uptakes in impaired mental functioning and movement.

Agitation is one of the most common effects of fear in dementias and Alzheimer's Disease. Agitation is generally expressed in combativeness and fidgeting or pacing.

Combativeness can be quite dangerous, so we need to ensure that the environment is safe for our loved ones and us. This means, in practical terms, removing actual weapons (guns, knives, etc.) and objects that could be used as weapons. Many times, our initial attempts to calm things down will temporarily increase combativeness, but it is important that we stay and be calm, and not get combative in return.

Gentle, non-threatening firmness, interestingly, will work in most situations because it brings our loved ones back into the present. It won't necessarily eradicate the fear, but it will usually stop the combativeness.

Fidgeting and pacing – the kind where our loved ones are compelled internally to move – is also very common as well.

A lot of healthy people unconsciously fidget when they're uncomfortable or stressed (the most common fidgeting behaviors are rocking back and forth, bouncing the legs and wringing the hands – if I'm sitting, I bounce my legs and have shaken more tables than I care to admit in my lifetime and if I'm standing, I rock back and forth), so to see fidgeting in our loved ones with dementias and Alzheimer's Disease should not surprise us.

What usually surprises us is there is nothing in the external environment that should be causing stress and/or fear, and since we don't know what's going on internally with our loved ones, we get blindsided by these behaviors.

A lot of healthy people also go "take a walk" to get calmed down during a stressful and/or fearful situation. I know I do. I've been a pacer all my life and I have to move – and move away from – stressful and/or fearful situations just to clear my head and be able to think things through and get calm.

Note: This different from "wandering," which has a specific intent in mind, and which we'll discuss in detail later in this book.

It's no different with our loved ones with dementias and Alzheimer's Disease, especially if they have been physically active all their lives. My mom was a walker and as these diseases progressed, she spent a lot of her waking time, day and night, walking. During the day, she'd walk outside. At night, she'd pace the halls.

The main concern for us is to make sure our loved ones are safe. The easiest way to do this is to walk with them as much as we're able to. Because one of the dementias that Mom had was Lewy Body dementia and because her panic and anxiety triggered TIA's, her precarious balance was one of the first visible physical signs I observed after I was consciously aware that she was having major neurological changes.

I will never forget the frightened phone call she made to me on a late winter day, a few months before we knew definitively what Mom's diagnosis was, to tell me that she'd been outside walking, and lost her balance and fell. Mom said she wasn't hurt and had only hit the back of her head on the grass, but she wanted me there at her retirement community. I went immediately, thankful, I was only five minutes away.

Mom was actually okay, but from that point on, I'd spend the bulk of the day there with her, and we'd take two or three walks around the property together with her holding onto my arm and me making sure she didn't lose her balance. Balance issues would be a concern the rest of her life.

3. Frustration
   We all know how we react when we want to do something, we know we should know how to do it, people keep saying "it's simple" and explaining it to us repeatedly, and we still can't make it happen.

   I'm like that with anything that requires me to listen to something and execute it simultaneously. It looks easy. I've tried to do it many times, even in public once in a beginner's aerobics class where I ended up stopping and walking out 30 seconds after the class began (and I didn't go back) because I simply could not do it the way everyone else was effortlessly doing it. I either have to listen fully, then execute, or I have to tune out all the noise and just do it on my own. I cannot do both at the same time.

   I get frustrated. Quickly. And eventually, I just gave up on any kind of exercise that forced me to have to listen and do at the same time. I'm a good athlete. But now I just do athletic things that don't force me to rely on being in sync with other people or having to follow instructions while trying to do it.

Now imagine how we would react if we found that things we've always done effortlessly, we know we should be able to continue to do them effortlessly, and well-meaning people remind us that they are simple to do, but even after repeated instructions, we couldn't do them?

That's the first prong of frustration with our loved ones suffering from dementias and Alzheimer's Disease: not being able to effortlessly do things they've always done. Repeated failures bring on frustration, and can, if not addressed kindly, patiently, and respectfully, lead to just giving up on trying them at all.

This is where the team approach I discussed in chapter 1 is so critical. By taking a "we" approach to common life activities with our loved ones, we can both ease the frustration and ensure that they don't just give up and quit altogether. Again, it takes time, patience, and gentleness, but it is worth it!

The second prong of frustration with our loved ones – and one that is the one that we just have to accept as current reality – is the partial or full inability to learn how to do anything new. Because dementias and Alzheimer's Disease affect short-term memory, it becomes impossible, at some point in these diseases, to acquire new skills and new knowledge.

My mom was always learning something new all her life. In her early 60's, I bought her a computer and printer and she, unlike my dad who said, "I used a typewriter all my life and I'll use a typewriter until I die" (in the last year of his life, Dad would sit beside Mom and read while she would type his stories and as they communicated with a congestive heart failure group online, a godsend for both of them, but Dad never touched the keyboard), eagerly jumped in and started learning how to use it.

Mom was slower at getting the terminology, but she stuck with it. When I got her online and showed her the internet and that we could email each other and save money on phone calls, she jumped into that too.

Mom took classes and watched videos for sign language and did fairly well learning to communicate in sign language, even getting me involved when we'd sit down for an hour or so every night and practice sign language together.

Mom loved learning and that was one of the passions of her life.

Because Mom had always been a bit fragmented about computer terminology, when I noticed her getting more frequently upset about things she couldn't remember or couldn't do, despite my clear, step-by-step notes for her, initially it didn't bother me.

However, as her dementias and Azheimer's Disease progressed and I became aware that some was changing neurologically, I saw frustration almost any time she sat down at the computer to do anything more than a Google search or an email.

Her frustration manifested itself in something I used to hate hearing her say - I believe it started in her childhood, when she already had a hearing loss that impacted her learning and speech, and it must have been something she heard enough to believe it when she couldn't do something - "I'm stupid."

(Ironically, hearing Mom say this about herself a lot during my life must have somehow worked itself way into my own response to failure or not being able to do something, because from the earliest time I remember, I have always thought or said "I'm stupid" or "I'm an idiot" when things go wrong or aren't working out, no matter what I do.

I get much, much harder on myself internally than I ever heard Mom express in her speech, but I wonder if she didn't think some of the same things about herself that I default to when I'm in the trenches fiercely fighting for just a fraction of forward movement and all I get is furthered bogged down where I'm standing.)

Mom was definitely very intelligent and would have never gone as far in life as she did without an excellent mind.

I would always reassure Mom that she wasn't stupid and that the things she was getting frustrated about were not a big deal in the big scheme of things. She'd dispute me for a while, but I stayed calm and just kept reassuring her until that moment of frustration was gone.

And I learned early on, before all of the neurological issues got front and center, that getting frustrated with frustration makes things worse. It's important to identify what is causing the frustration and figuring out how to eliminate it, instead of reacting with frustration ourselves.

Sometimes the simplest things can be a source of frustration for our loved ones suffering with dementias and Alzheimer's Disease. If we can find out what the source is, then we can work on eliminating the frustration.

And the need for calm reassurance and a gentle, loving touch, over and over, cannot be overstated. Again, it takes patience, time, and self-control, but we have responsibility to calm the flames instead of adding fuel to the fire.

4. Anger

Anger is another common reaction to fear and/or stress. It is one of the strongest defense mechanisms we as humans have. The need to lash out at someone else comes from our own discomfort in our selves. Part of the reason is that when we're feeling bad, we want other people to feel bad.

This is never a conscious decision, even in those of us who are healthy, but the difference between us and our loved ones with neurological damage is that we still have intact control mechanisms in our brains to know that, in general, anger just isn't the appropriate response most of the time, and if anger is the appropriate response, then there is a right and wrong way and right and wrong time to express it.

In our loved ones suffering from dementias and Alzheimer's Disease, because the brain is compromised by damage to impulse control and sound executive judgment, the filters aren't there anymore to stop the anger at the gate of the brain and the mouth before it comes out.

Additionally, there is no concept of right and wrong ways to express anger, so whatever our loved ones are experiencing comes out, often without warning, in a full-tilt, unedited, and all-out assault.

Mom had a lot of anger early in life (her childhood was a nightmare in so many ways) and always had a temper, but as we kids were growing up, she worked very hard – not without some failures – to control, master, and, significantly eliminate them.

By the time Mom was in her early 60's, she seemed to have worked through most of her anger and had mellowed considerably. There were still flashes from time to time of her temper and her anger, but they were usually when she felt protective of her family.

After Dad died, Mom seemed to mellow even more. She could still rip you apart if the circumstances were right, but it was so rare by then that it had all but disappeared off the grid of who she was.

Then, out of nowhere, the anger started popping up unexpectedly about the time Mom was in the beginning stages of mild cognitive impairment (this is hindsight recognizing this because it sure threw me for a loop at the time). It wasn't often, but, looking back, it coincided with times when she believed she wasn't wanted around (not true, but no reasoning with what she had in her mind) or she misheard or misconstrued or completely made up something I said or she thought I said.

As Mom's neurological damage progressed, still undetectable in most situations, her angry episodes coincided mainly with and during hospitalizations. But as she was moving into the middle stages of dementias and Alzheimer's Disease, the episodes of anger escalated until just before we were able to get her on the right medications to control the behaviors, Mom was on the warpath all the time.

I absolutely hate conflict and anger, whether it's directed at me or not, because my response to it is panic and anxiety. My first instinct is always to just get away from it as fast as I can when it starts and either stay away for good or give the situation a long cooling period to ensure it's over.

But I realized that Mom's anger was really fear because she knew something was wrong, but she didn't know what was wrong, so I would stay – not for a long time – and take it and reassure her that I wasn't going anywhere and that I loved her.

Again, reassurance and love repeatedly expressed and demonstrated with our loved ones with dementias and Alzheimer's Disease, are the best ways to deal with anger.

It's important as well for us not to engage, as hard as that may be. It can be tempting and it can be hard for us not to. But this is where we must exercise self-control.

It is our responsibility to be calm, to be the voices of reason, to be the peacemakers, no matter how intense our loved ones' anger is.

They don't know what they are doing, but we do, and while they're not responsible for their behavior, we are totally responsible for ours.

The next step in the journey of the neurological changes that occur with dementias and Alzheimer's Disease appear in communicating: speaking, writing, reading, and hearing.

At this point, it's probably a good idea to look at the major regions of the brain and see why the neurological damage tends to follow the same pattern in the same sequence. The progression of these steps mirror that sequence.

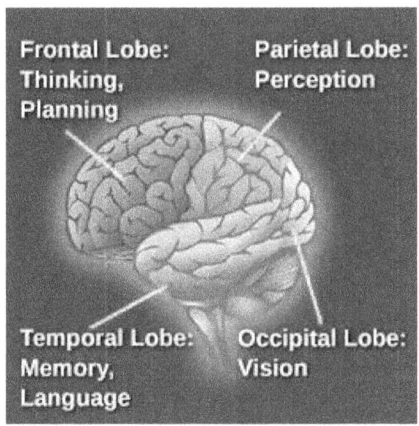

Mild cognitive impairment generally occurs because of neurological damage to the outer layers of the frontal lobe of the brain and the temporal lobe of the brain, and, in the case of Alzheimer's Disease, which refers to the "tangles and plaque" shrinkage of the brain due to brain-cell death, these are the first places in the brain where cells begin to die.

As more cells die, the functions that these areas of the brain control become more profoundly affected. Language function is controlled in a deeper portion of the temporal lobe, so in the case of just Alzheimer's Disease, communication problems might not show up for a while.

However, if our loved ones are suffering from other dementias, such as vascular dementia which causes clusters of cell death through the brain, even the innermost parts, because of a stroke or chronic small-vessel ischemia (usually the result of mini-strokes or transient ischemic attacks, also known as TIA's), then communication problems may occur sooner.

Regardless of how long it takes, communication problems are the third definitive step in the journey, whether it's a short step or a longer step.

Communication problems in dementias and Alzheimer's Disease include fall under the general term of aphasia.

Aphasia is simply neurological impairment that affects language. This impairment can be mild, moderate, or severe, and affects speaking, reading, writing, and comprehension of words. Depending on the progression rates and types of dementias our loved ones are suffering from, the degree of aphasia may or may not change dramatically. It really depends on time and the extent of neurological deterioration in the temporal lobe of the brain.

The severity of aphasia is very individualized, so although it's a step in dementias and Alzheimer's Disease, our loved ones will not necessarily experience it exactly the same way. Additionally, our loves ones with dementias and

Alzheimer's Disease may not experience each type of aphasia to the same extent and each type may materialize at different stages in these neurological diseases.

There are four broad categories of aphasia:

1. Expressive aphasia

    Expressive aphasia is also known as non-fluent aphasia (Broca's aphasia, which results from damage to the Broca area of the frontal lobe, most often as the result of a stroke, is a form of expressive aphasia).

    Temporary (lasting for less than one hour) expressive aphasia can occur as a result of migraines and transient ischemic attacks (TIA's).

    In expressive aphasia, our loved ones know exactly what they want to say or write, but they have great difficulty actually doing it. However, they are usually able to understand what they hear or read.

    Expressive aphasia is characterized by agrammatism (the inability to form complete or intelligible sentences while being able to articulate single words) which includes halting and garbled or incomplete speech and writing.

    This is most often in the form of a disconnected string of words that excludes relational words for action (verbs), relationship (prepositions and conjunctions), and specification (pronouns, articles, particles, and adverbs).

But, instead of boring you with a review of the grammatical parts of speech here, the easiest way to describe what gets omitted in expressive aphasia sentences is to say they are the descriptor words that give context and meaning.

A simple example would be "House..........cat............doctor." This means very little of and by itself.

However, there is a two-fold approach that we need to use to encourage our loved ones to communicate as long as they are able and to make sure our loved ones are understood.

The first approach is to resist the urges to hurry our loved ones along as they strive to express themselves or to assume we know what they mean and use our own words to fill in the gaps.

We've all probably, at some point, been in the situation where we were trying to simultaneously formulate and verbalize a thought or idea and gotten stuck as we were trying to find, let's say, a diplomatic way of saying something so we wouldn't be misunderstood or would not cause offense, and the people we were talking to jumped in and finished it for us – inaccurately and not even remotely close to what we were actually going to say – before we had time to find the words.

Do you remember that frustration? And do you remember what happened as a result of that frustration? You quit talking and made a promise to yourself to avoid trying to communicate at any length with that person ever again.

That will happen with our loved ones with expressive aphasia as well if we constantly rush them – giving the impression that we don't have time for them – and try to fill in the gaps for them – putting words in their mouths. Because they know exactly what they want to say or write, these two things will lead to constant frustration and shutdown.

So the second approach we need to take is to invest the time with our loved ones to find out what the missing words are. In the sentence above, "house," "cat," and "doctor" are our only clues. So we have a little detective work to do.

If all the words in the sentence are applicable to our loved one, then it's time to start asking simple questions (ones with "yes" and "no" answers are the easiest to answer) until we can figure out what our loved ones are trying to communicate to us about the house, the cat, and the doctor.

I'll give an example of the kind of questions I'd ask. "Does the cat need its shots?" "Is the cat sick?" "Has the cat been staying inside or outside the house more?" "Do you want me to schedule an appointment for us to take the cat to the vet?"

Based on those three words, that's the first conclusion I would draw, but the questions help our loved ones communicate effectively and, more importantly, to be heard. And questions include them in the communication process, which encourages continued communication, which is always the goal for as long as our loved ones are able to communicate.

2. Receptive aphasia

   Receptive aphasia (also known as Wernicke's aphasia, fluent aphasia, and sensory aphasia) exists when our loved ones can still express themselves in speech, they can still hear and read, but they are not be able comprehend what they hear or read.

   Neurological damage to the medial section of the temporal lobe (where the Wernicke's area is located) is responsible for receptive aphasia, and because of the location of the damage, the occipital (vision), parietal (perception), and temporal (memory and language) regions from the core language center of the brain are affected.

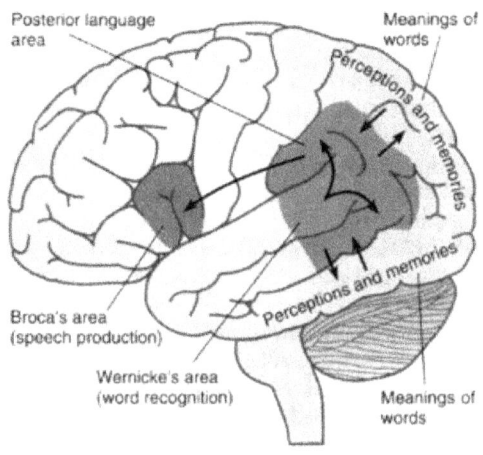

Our loved ones with receptive aphasia lose both comprehension and context of language, even though they generally are able to speak using normal grammar, syntax, and inflexion. Because of the lack of access to the normal input (reception) and output (expression) synergy of conversation, communication usually ends up resembling two trains on different tracks going in opposite directions.

What we plan to speak meaningfully begins in the Wernicke's area of the brain. Once the plan is completed, it is then transmitted to the Broca's area of the brain. With receptive aphasia, the ability to plan speech is lost, as is the comprehension of words that are spoken or written.

Ironically, our loved ones with receptive aphasia will often become very talkative, but everything they say will be random as far as context. It's important to be aware that our loved ones not only don't understand external input (speech and reading), but they also don't understand the meaning of what they are saying.

The main reason this happens is because our loved ones with receptive aphasia lose the ability to categorize sounds. Because so many words either sound the same (hail, hell, and hale, for example) or similar (pin and pen and hill and heel, for example), the damage to the Wernicke's area of the brain removes that fine-tuning of categorization that enables our loved ones to isolate significant sound characteristics and translate them into something meaningful.

In spite of this, however, there are some very effective strategies for successfully communicating with our loved ones with receptive aphasia.

One is to keep our speech slow and simple. Because of the difficulty in distinguishing between significant sounds and categorizing them meaningfully, the more rapid and the more complex our speech is, the less likely our loved ones will understand what we are saying. Slowing down and enunciating our speech may help with comprehension.

Repeat information simply, without being condescending or shouting – remember, it's not that they can't hear, but they can't comprehend – and try to confirm comprehension before moving on in the conversation.

We can also use gestures to add meaning to speech. For example, if we want to ask if our loved ones are cold, we could hug ourselves and shiver. If we want to ask them if they're hungry, we could use the motion of eating, or if they're thirsty, the motion of drinking.

Because images get processed in a different part of the brain than speech and writing, we can also use "props" to communicate as well, either in the form of drawing or simply by getting the item we're talking about and showing it to our loved ones.

An example of this would be getting a sweater or blanket and showing our loved ones that to see if they're cold. For eating and drinking questions, it would include actually getting food and drink out and handing it to our loved ones to see whether they accept it or refuse it.

Interestingly enough, our loved ones with expressive aphasia will often resort to gestures to communicate as well, so it's important to be engaged so we don't miss crucial gestures that could tell us what our loved ones are really trying to communicate.

There are other things to we need to utilize for effective communication with our loved ones with receptive aphasia.

One is to limit blocks of communication to one subject. This can help keep confusion to a minimum and can also improve the communication process. Another is to break communication and tasks into steps and present and complete one step at a time. This will eliminate a lot of frustration.

3. Anomic aphasia

Anomic aphasia (also known as dysnomia, nominal aphasia, and amnesiac aphasia) refers to difficulty recalling or finding the right word – even though our loved ones know the right word - when speaking and writing.

In this form of aphasia, our loved ones often speak circuitously as they're trying to find the right word or they use the wrong word (usually something close in sound to the right word). This same close-to-the-right-word selection is evident in our loved ones' writing too.

Anomic aphasia is generally seen in three areas of communication: word selection (inability to find the right word), semantic deficit (inability to both name and recognize objects), and disconnection anomia (inability to accurately name and recognize objects in all sensory contexts: for example, our loved ones might be able to accurately identify a cup when they see a cup, but do not know what a cup is when they hear the word "cup").

Anomic aphasia occurs because of damage to both the parietal and temporal lobes of the brain. It is most commonly seen in our loved ones who have suffered strokes and who suffer from vascular dementia, as this form of aphasia is cause by the death of cells in clusters and affects how information flows through the pathways of the brain.

Think of a highway taking us from point A to point B. The trip is five miles and should take us no more than 15 minutes. Imagine that two miles after we've gotten on the highway, there's a major accident and traffic is being detoured to the exit just before where the accident occurred.

Now we have to figure out where we are and then find a new way through a route we don't usually take to get to point B. That takes time, but we start on the new route toward our destination of point B, which will get us to our destination in 15 minutes.

However, we've lost time with the accident and the detour and having to recalculate a new route in less familiar surroundings, so we're already running late.

Now, while we're on the detour route, we encounter road work that takes us off the detour route and onto a new route. Once again, we have to try to find a new way to get to point B, and that is assuming we even know where we are in relationship to point B on the new route.

This takes even more time as we have to start all over figuring out how to get to point B. This time the route gets us there, but instead of five miles and 15 minutes, we've had to drive 20 miles and it's taken us 45 minutes to get to point B.

That's a pretty close analogy of what happens in the brain with anomic aphasia.

The most effective strategies for communicating with our loved ones with anomic aphasia are patience, listening, and asking the right questions. Since our loved ones know what they are trying to communicate, but can't find the correct word, they will often resort to describing it (this is called circumlocution) in their communication.

A simple example of this would be "It's round. You know that thing that you put on a pan. It keeps things from boiling over." The answer, of course, is a "lid." We would go get the lid and show it to our loved one and get confirmation that's what he or she is talking about.

For the more complex descriptions, it's important to use both questions and the actual item(s) we think our loved ones may be talking about. Most of the time, seeing the right object will be enough to move the communication process along. However, sometimes, it will just take time, patience, and very attuned listening to understand what our loved ones are talking about.

4. Global aphasia

Global aphasia affects all types of communications and can range from simply recognizing personal names (children, spouses, grandchildren) when our loved ones hear them, but not being able to say the names, to being able to make partial sounds, to being unable to speak at all.

Most incidences of global aphasia in our loved ones are the result of large middle-cerebral-artery strokes, which affect all the language-processing areas of the brain. This includes the ability to comprehend and speak or write.

However, there still can be some effective ways of communicating with our loved ones with global aphasia.

The first is to use touch to get their attention and to connect with them. Touch is one the most powerful forms of communication and can often stand alone in the absence of words.

The second is to use simple gestures and facial expressions to communicate. Much of what we think and feel ends up showing up in our body language – which is often how we determine whether a person is being honest with us when either their words and body language match or they do not – so we can use this to convey our messages to our loved ones.

The third way to communicate with our loved ones with global aphasia is by using simple language and giving them time to respond, without rushing them or jumping in and trying to guess what they are trying to say in response.

Hallucinations, both visual and auditory, are commonly the next step in the journey of dementias and Alzheimer's Disease. Visual hallucinations are generally more prevalent than auditory hallucinations, and can include people – usually loved ones – who are dead or nondescript strangers.

In my mom's case, one hallucination led her to ask me "Do you see those two angels over there?," as she pointed toward a bookcase across the room from the couch where we were sitting (I didn't, but I asked her to tell me about what she was seeing).

Although some of these hallucinations may provoke anxiety and fear, often, especially in the case of seeing long-lost loved ones, they are as comforting as they are real to our loved ones. I remember the first time my mom told me that my dad, who'd been dead for 12 years, had come to visit her the night before and then proceeded to tell me all about their conversations and how good it was to see him. Then Mom said he'd left just before I came into the room.

Well-formed and insightful hallucinations (either manifestations of things and/or people who are not there or the perception that still objects are moving) are overwhelmingly prevalent in our loved ones suffering from Lewy Body dementia, where Lewy bodies are present in the temporal area of the brain (particularly in the amygdala and parahippocampal regions).

LIMBIC SYSTEM STRUCTURES

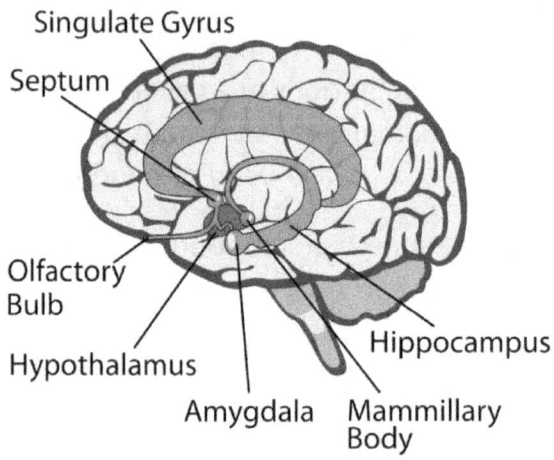

The amygdala is linked to aggression and emotions, and is involved in emotional learning, forming long-term memories, and the hormone secretion (along with the pituitary gland) that tells the adrenal glands to release the copious amounts of adrenaline associated with the "flight-or-fight" response to fear, anxiety, and panic.

The parahippocampal (surrounding the hippocampus) region of the brain is responsible for encoding and retrieving memories of landscapes and scenery (faces and facial recognition happens in the fusiform gyrus region of the brain).

Early hallucinations are often seen in short-lived episodes of delirium that are triggered by stress (hospitalizations are the most frequent source of this kind of stress and the subsequent episodes of delirium).

Delirium can be exhibited by actual hallucinations. My mom spent her first full day in ICU in the late summer of 2008 (she was admitted after her blood pressure and heart rate crashed just a few hours after being sent home from the ER, in spite of my repeated advocacy for admission and my written objection that Mom wasn't admitted, because of an incompetent ER doctor who insisted on giving her round of after round of blood-pressure-lowering medication in response to Mom's abnormally high blood pressure) and started the day around 7 a.m. with a rambling, nonsensical conversation with her cardiologist and me.

I wound up having to answer the questions the cardiologist was asking because Mom was clearly not in the same room or conversation with us. I'd never seen delirium and I'd never seen Mom like that, so I was completely confused as to what was going on.

My sister, who came in from out of town a couple of hours later, and I sat with Mom all day and into the night, until we weren't allowed to stay anymore. Looking back, I'm not really sure now if Mom really knew us most of that day. We were uninitiated so it wasn't a question that would have occurred to either of us then.

Mom was in a good mood, but around 9:30 that morning, she pointed out to the nurses' station and said "Look! They're having a party and eating cake." My sister and I both looked and no one was at the nurses' station. Some form of that conversation went on most of the morning. While Mom was eating lunch, her mind darkened suddenly and briefly and she, without any provocation, laid into my sister with the statement, "Don't look at me with that look of hate!"

Then the darkness was gone almost as suddenly and the rest of the afternoon was spent with Mom asking us if we could see the letters up in the air above her bed, as she traced them with her fingers and "read" them out loud, and then more activity at the nurses' station with plane crashes and wildlife intermixed. None of this seemed to disturb Mom, but she gave us an almost-non-stop blow-by-blow account of what she was seeing.

Although this was disturbing to both of us, my sister and I finally accepted that nothing was there and quit looking each time Mom pointed and just listened and asked her questions about what she was seeing.

By dinnertime, the delirium had stopped and Mom got dark again, and then got agitated (which is normal as well).

There were two more instances of delirium with Mom during that hospitalization. One occurred the next night when she was finally alert after a day of mostly non-responsiveness and she accused me of putting her in a nursing home without discussing it with her. Another occurred a few days later when she was convinced she was in a mental hospital.

Then, after Mom's release, as far as I know, it stopped.

I didn't see it again until the next hospitalization almost a year later, in the summer of 2009, after Mom had pacemaker surgery, when she was convinced that she had been kidnapped was being held against her will and wanted me to call the police to come rescue her.

Again, after Mom's release, as far as I was aware, it stopped for a few months, but began again, this time in earnest and more frequently in the fall of that year.

By this time, it was slowly dawning on me that Mom was seeing things that did not happen and people who were not there, because by now paranoia (which we'll discuss in the next chapter) was beginning to come to the forefront, as well as an aggressiveness and argumentativeness that I hadn't ever seen before.

That autumn, at least once a week, Mom would tell me that someone else – with whom Mom had begun to have a particularly contentious relationship, despite the two of them having known each other in a friendly way for seven years – at her retirement community was coming into her room and stealing things.

Mom told me she walked in and caught this lady one day in the act of theft and they argued and the lady left.

At the same time, things in Mom's apartment started habitually going missing and Mom blamed this lady. I had the locks changed and three keys made: one for me, one for Mom, and one for the community manager. I gave the community manager instructions that no one be allowed into Mom's apartment unless one of the three of us were present. She agreed and Mom seemed satisfied with that.

However, the escalation of tensions and accusations between Mom and the lady she accused of breaking into her place got worse by the day. These two were at war with each other by then.

And, once again, Mom said she saw this lady going in and out of her room. Some paperwork that we needed went missing and Mom immediately accused this lady of stealing it. I spent a few hours one day methodically going through all of Mom's paperwork and found this missing paperwork in the wrong folder of a locked organizer that Mom kept in her apartment.

I told Mom I'd found it and that the lady she thought took it from her did not and that she needed to apologize to the lady for accusing her of theft.

Whether Mom ever apologized, I don't know. But she continued to insist that this lady was breaking into her apartment and stealing things.

Within two or three months, as 2010 began, Mom began to see Daddy on a regular basis. Until then, she'd mentioned seeing him maybe once or twice a year. Daddy always came to see Mom when I was not there and he always left just before I got there. Mom would tell me in detail about the conversations they had and how glad she was to see Daddy again.

By the early spring of 2010, Mom began having regular hallucinations. SeroquelXR effectively eliminated Mom's hallucinations until, because of her Lewy Body dementia, in late November 2011, she developed late-stage tardive dyskinesia because of the antipsychotic, and we had to discontinue it. Mom's hallucinations came back within a month, but other than one instance of some anxiety they did not seem to create fear in her.

Hallucinations fall into the visuoperceptual changes that occur as neurological damage affects how the brain handles vision and perception.

The causes can be actual damage to the brain (lesions and seizures are primarily responsible for this), the disturbance of neurotransmitter chemistry, and the transition of subconscious thinking into conscious thinking.

Hallucinations, whether a result of one or a combination of these neurological factors, are a real and sometimes difficult-to-manage part of the journeys our loved ones with dementias and Alzheimer's Disease go through.

In the early emergence of hallucinations, it is common to have both fear and comfort as a by-product of the hallucinations.

Fear is generally expressed because of the presence of strangers our loved one sees as part of their hallucinations.

It may be a recurring stranger or group of strangers – for my mom, it was a boy and a girl who walked into her apartment every time she walked out and left just as she was coming back in and a man who walked into her bathroom every day and straightened up the towel and washcloth she had hanging on the towel rack.

She was afraid of them, not because she believed they were going to physically harm her, but because she believed they were stealing and hiding things from her.

Mom's comfort in her hallucinations was with the ones that involved Daddy. I know Mama missed him terribly all of those years since his death in 1998, and I believe the last few years of her life that Daddy being back in her life gave her an anchor that she'd been missing.

The most important thing to remember with hallucinations – and I had to learn this with Mom – is that just because they are not real to us doesn't mean they're not real to our loved ones with dementias and Alzheimer's Disease. Dismissing them, ridiculing them, or scolding our loved ones with statements like "C'mon, you know that's not real!" is not the right way to handle hallucinations.

The best way to handle them – and especially to find out what's going on behind them (there's a reason for them occurring) and to eliminate or manage any hallucinations that might create fear, panic, or anxiety in our loved ones – is to listen and to talk about them with our loved ones.

Often, hallucinations are the product of long-term memories in the subconscious – especially related to family and friends who were loved deeply – becoming conscious and, for our loved ones, becoming real. It's as though the movies in the their minds are suddenly being projected in front of them as if they're actually taking place in real time.

By listening to our loved ones talk through what they're seeing, we can learn a lot about what's on their mind and, sometimes, the things they miss and the things they long for and the things they believe they need to make peace with.

When we listen to them, ask questions, and learn more, we have an opportunity to connect with our loved ones where they are instead of imposing where we are on them.

Chapter 5: "Confusion Never Stops, Closing Walls and Ticking Clocks"

Pervasive paranoia is the next step in the journey of dementias and Alzheimer's Disease. At some point, hallucinations and paranoia tend to overlap – the hallucinations, especially if they're scary will elicit panic and anxiety – but paranoia eventually stands on its own as a distinct step in the journey.

Paranoia has a complicated root system that we'll break down into its components so that we understand why it occurs and what it looks like.

1. One of the roots of paranoia in our loved ones with dementias and Alzheimer's Disease is confusion and fear. There is self-awareness, at this point, within our loved ones that something is really wrong. They don't know what it is, but the feedback around them, spoken and unspoken, tells them that they can't trust themselves.

   Persistent hallucinations leave them with blurred lines between what's real and what's not. Constant corrections to the information our loved ones believe is true creates widening doubt. Repeated proofs that disprove what our loved ones believe to be accurate create insecurity.

   All of this also creates anger and fear because humans are wired to trust themselves – their reasoning, their assessments, their intuitions, their processing of the external world – more than to trust any other human being. When that innate ability is constantly challenged and proven faulty, it's scary and it is infuriating.

The normal reaction is to fall back to a protective position that rejects everybody else and defends the self. Paranoia is the result.

2. Another root of paranoia is an increasingly-damaged neurological network that can no longer provide our loved ones with reliable and trustworthy input. Everything that can be perceived through the five senses of vision, hearing, touch, taste, and smell has been altered. These are basic functions of human life and when they fail then nothing in the physical world can be trusted.

3. A third root of paranoia is experience, personality, and temperament. The more basic trust issues that our loved ones have experienced in their lives, whether in childhood, adulthood, or old age (or a combination of all three), the more these will contribute to increasing paranoia with dementias and Alzheimer's Disease.

Additionally, the more anxious and fearful, as well as the more naturally-suspicious, our loved ones have been because of personality and temperament throughout life, the greater impact this will have on the level of paranoia they experience and exhibit.

One of the common areas of paranoia among our loved ones with dementias and Alzheimer's Disease is the belief that everybody is stealing - or trying to steal - everything from them. The primary focus is financial, but it applies to everything else in our loved ones' lives.

Why?

1. Our loved ones are most often on a fixed income, with savings, retirement, and possibly government pensions (such as Social Security in the United States). That is limited financial security for our loved ones - since they have no ability to earn any more - and they tend to be hyperconscious of the finiteness of it.

    Therefore, when they start misplacing cash, they immediately assume it's been stolen. What actually happens is that as their paranoia about theft increases, so does the need to hide everything in a "safe place" where nobody can find it. The problem is that with short-term memory loss also accelerating, they forget what "safe place" they moved it to and when they can't find it, then it's been stolen from them.

    The other area of finances that our loved ones' paranoia extends to is that of handling their financial matters (paying bills, banking accounts, etc.). As we step in to help our loved ones with their financial matters, it tangibly, even though they ask us for help and need our help, takes full control away from them to some degree and makes us prime targets for accusations of theft.

With my mom, we had a living revocable trust set up (her idea) that would give me access to her financial accounts to do business for her in the case of her death or if she was not competent to handle it herself.

My name was never on any of her bank accounts and I never had access to her financials until her breakdown in the summer of 2010 when I had to pay her bills (I kept detailed financial records and paid everything with her checks and her credit card/bank account, unless, as I'd done over the years, I was financially helping her out).

I realize now that Mom didn't really understand that me sitting down and helping her with the bills and financials didn't mean I had carte blanche assess to her money. She didn't understand that my being able to log in to her bank account online didn't mean I had the authority to spend the money. The lines were already blurred for her.

And as her paranoia increased, the accusations that I was stealing her money, only wanted her money, and wanted her out of the way so I could have her money increased as well.

Not completely realizing where Mom was in the dementias and Alzheimer's Disease journey, every time an accusation was leveled, I patiently and calmly explained to Mom that none of that was true: I didn't have the ability and I'd rather have her than whatever small amount of money she had left to take care of her.

I'd say the same thing I said to her every time we talked about finances after my dad died: "Mama, Daddy left that money to take care of you. It's not mine and if it's all gone the day you die and the check I write to the funeral home bounces (it didn't, by the way, because I paid what the small burial policy didn't cover), then it was spent the way Daddy wanted it to be spent."

It didn't change anything. In fact, it usually elicited more anger and more yelling at me. I learned to say it once each time and then be quiet.

Mom's paranoia about her finances escalated to the point that in the two months before her breakdown – and the right diagnoses and medications – I was taking to her to the bank almost every day.

Mom wouldn't let me go in with her. She'd go in, stay for a while, and then come back to the car. She'd get in, glare at me, and furtively stuff a little piece of paper with handwriting on it into her purse.

Later, when I cleaned out Mom's purse, I found all those little strips of paper with her bank account balances written on them, unchanged except for the few dollars she was spending each day when I took her to the grocery store or the drug store to buy one or two things.

Mom probably told the bank I was stealing money from her, but they knew that not only was I not stealing money from Mom, but I couldn't steal money from her. However, Mom also told the director at the independent retirement community where she was living that I was stealing money from her. The director reported it to Adult Protective Services, who had begun an investigation into whether I was stealing money from Mom.

I found this out two days before Mom was hospitalized in the geriatric psychiatric hospital and provided the director with a full financial record for Mom for the time period Mom was accusing me of stealing money from her, and as soon as the director reviewed it, she said "you've helped your mom with her money and you've done a good job." She said she would call Adult Protective Services and call off the investigation. I never heard anything else about it.

In addition, on at least two occasions, Mom tried to have me arrested for stealing her money. There may have been – and probably were – even more, but I know only about the two.

One occurred one night when Mom walked from her apartment down to an Armed Forces recruiting station in a shopping center not far from her. Mom must have thought they were the police.

According to the hospital, when I got called inside by their security after Mom had me stop there one day to "get paperwork," the Armed Forces recruiting office called an ambulance to take Mom to the hospital for a full physical and mental evaluation, as well as a toxicology screen, which lasted most of the night, and the hospital released her and sent her home the next morning around 6:30 am.

This was the first I knew anything about that hospital visit. However, Mom had told my sister a couple of weeks early that she was in the hospital around the same time, but on a different night.

I told my sister at the time that Mom had just imagined it (although I couldn't figure out why). But she didn't imagine it. It happened. No one called me either from the hospital or the retirement community where Mom lived and to this day, I have absolutely no idea how Mom got home that morning.

The second time Mom called the police to arrest me for stealing her money was the afternoon of the day my sister said Mom told her she'd been in the hospital the night before.

I'd already spent most of the morning with Mom and she seemed fine when I left. My sister, during our phone call where we both agreed that Mom needed some psychiatric help but neither of us had any idea how to make it happen, suggested I go check on Mom again.

When I arrived and pulled into a parking space, I noticed that a running police cruiser was in the space to the left of mine. My stomach immediately knotted up and I somehow instinctively knew that Mom had called the police.

I got out of the car and walked to the front door where I was met by a staff nurse. Over her shoulder I could see the cop and hear Mom. I asked what happened. The nurse realized I was Mom's daughter, so she stood in front of me so that Mom could not see me and said "let's wait until they go back to your mom's apartment and then we can talk."

Mom and the cop went to Mom's apartment and the nurse and I walked in and sat down. The nurse said that Mom had called 911 and wanted to cops to come out and arrest me. We talked for a while and I explained the situation with Mom and the nurse took my hand and held it briefly and said "I know. I understand. It will be okay."

About 15 minutes later, Mom and the cop came back to the door. Mom saw me and hugged me. I asked the cop if everything was okay and he said, "Yes, she just needed to talk and she's okay now." I thanked him and he told me he had a mother too, so it was no problem.

When I went back to Mom's apartment with her, she started crying and hugged me and told me she was sorry and she knew I loved her and was helping her. I held her close for a long time, tears in my own eyes because I couldn't fix this and, more than anything else in the world, I wanted to, reassuring her that it was okay and I loved her always and unconditionally.

That is often how the tenor of paranoia rises and wanes, so don't be surprised when one minute our loved ones are raging at us or to someone else about us and the next they are sorrowful and telling us they love us. Both things are true.

2. The second part of paranoia about theft involves things. As our loved ones with dementias and Alzheimer's Disease increasingly misplace items, in part because of short-term memory loss, and in part because they move them around a lot (this is a side effect of the paranoia) and then don't remember where they "hid" them to keep them safe from theft, the more our loved ones believe everyone else is stealing from them.

    And they will accuse us and everyone else of stealing from them without hesitation. Put simply, if our loved ones can't find something, then it was stolen.

    The last thing Mom accused me of stealing before she was hospitalized and properly medicated was a three-ring-binder she kept her bank statements in.

    I looked everywhere in that apartment – the oven, the freezer, the refrigerator, the cabinet in the bathroom, under her mattress, you name it, I looked – for that notebook and couldn't find it. All the while, she was telling me I needed to get out because she'd called the police and they were coming to arrest me.

I finally gave up and left, not totally sure that the police weren't on their way to arrest me because Mom was so angry and so sure I had come in during the night and stolen that notebook.

Two days later, after she'd called 911 at 3:30 that morning and they'd taken her to the hospital for another psych evaluation and at 7:15 that morning I'd agreed to have her committed to a geriatric psychiatric hospital, I went to Mom's apartment to pack a bag to take to the hospital that afternoon for her.

I decided to clean up while I was there. In the process of cleaning, I walked over to the part of the room where Mom had been sitting and accusing me of stealing two days earlier. I hadn't gone anywhere near her that day. I happened to turn around and diagonally across from me, behind the one dresser I had not looked behind, was the three-ring-binder that Mom had accused me of stealing.

I sighed and shook my head. What else could I do? You'll sigh and shake your head a lot too. What else can you do?

The irony, perhaps, of paranoia is that the closer our relationships to our loved ones, the more frequently and viciously we will be the target of the accusations that arise from paranoia.

You might as well expect this because it will happen. And it is hard to withstand well over the long haul. However, we must withstand it, not respond to the accusations, and stay calm, level-headed and unemotional throughout the course of paranoia's rampant run with our loved ones with dementias and Alzheimer's Disease.

Nobody else in the room is fully neurologically functional at the moment but us, so the burden for handling it the right way falls solely on us.

There are several important facets of handling this as well as possible (you can't manage it, because paranoia tells our loved ones we can't be trusted, so they won't believe anything we say, and you just have to accept that).

1. Try to find a solution to what's "missing," if the paranoia is about theft. The more concrete evidence of things not being stolen we can give, the more, even if it's just temporary, peace of mind our loved ones with dementias and Alzheimer's Disease will have.

2. Stay emotionally neutral. We can laugh or cry or both when we're by ourselves, but emotional neutrality with our loved ones is critical to not escalating their fears.

3. Stay calm. If we're not excited about anything, we can sometimes take the wind out of the sails of our loved ones' excitability. It's imperative for us to keep a calm

expression and to keep our voices and our tones calm. Because we're dealing with a person whose input comprehension has become faulty, everything that we say or do or express has the opportunity to be misinterpreted. We have to make sure that we don't do anything to help that opportunity along.

4. Don't argue, don't defend, and don't scream and yell back. This takes a lot of self-control, especially when we know what we're being accused of is completely untrue. But because we're not dealing with accurate reason, perception, or facts, we have to resist the urge to come back at them full force.

   In many ways, this self-control resembles what adults should do with children who are upset because they don't fully understand, perceive, and know all the facts. It's not right to lash out with all we've got at children when they simply aren't mature enough and haven't lived long enough to know what we know.

   The same principle, in reverse, applies to our loved ones with dementias and Alzheimer's Disease. They've lost what we still have and it's not right for us to lash out at them because, through no fault of their own, they don't understand anymore.

   I think this is one of the greatest gifts we can give our loved ones. I know personally how hard it can be to do.

Sometimes it took a lot of saying "you can't do this" to myself, counting to 10, big sighing, clenching my jaws to keep my mouth shut, and cheek and tongue-biting for me to do it.

But we have to do. The alternative is unacceptable. It's a character-builder, for sure, and the more we do it, the easier it becomes.

And an interesting and a good side effect will be a whole lot more empathy and more compassion, not just for our loved ones, but for humanity in general.

Dramatic and sudden mood swings are part and parcel of the journey through dementias and Alzheimer's Disease, and they begin to materialize during the step of paranoia, but they can continue throughout the course of these diseases.

There can be several triggers for these mood swings: environmental, physiological, perceptual, and neurological. Sometimes all of these can be in play at the same time, but normally the trigger is singular.

Let's take a look at each of the areas that can trigger a mood swing in our loved ones suffering with dementias and Alzheimer's Disease and how we can respond to and/or eliminate them.

1. Environmental changes are often the trigger for sudden and dramatic mood swings. These can include something as seemingly simple as moving something out of a familiar place or having our loved ones in a setting they are not familiar with. It can also include the presence of strangers (or people they don't remember) and it can include being asked to do something new or unfamiliar.

   For example, one of the most common instances of these kinds of mood swings is with medical personnel. Most nurses, nurse practioners, physician's assistants, and doctors have stories about routine care they were providing for a patient with dementias and Alzheimer's Disease that quickly deteriorated into yelling, screaming, aggression, and sometimes even physical assault.

The problem (and a lot of medical personnel are oblivious to this, not because they want to be, but because they see so many patients every day, it doesn't occur to them that being new to a person with dementias and Alzheimer's Disease would send that person into distress and trigger the mood swing), however, is not with the examinations or medical care, per se, but with the change in the people involved in that care.

I remember the day the home health agency sent a different nurse to our house for Mom's checkup and blood work. Not only was the nurse disorganized (she called me to schedule her visit when she was five minutes from the house; our regular nurse called first thing in the morning to set her appointment time for the day) and incompetent (she tried to draw blood twice and simply couldn't get it right, but wanted to try a third time – that got nixed in short order because the nurse was inept and Mom was not a happy camper at all by then), but she was not the regular nurse, and it sent Mom into a tailspin mood-wise.

To compound matters, the home health agency decided to send yet another nurse later the same afternoon to try to do the blood draw again (I gave that nurse a "one-and-done" limit up front) and that made it even harder on Mom and her mood reflected that.

It's important to realize that any disruptions to an established routine are environmental changes that will likely trigger a mood swing in our loved ones.

These kinds of disruptions are the ones that we have the most ability to minimize, if not eliminate altogether. How?

It's important for us to lead our loved ones' care teams and part of that means ensuring as much continuity in those involved on the team as is humanly possible. When we started home health care, I asked that the same nurse and physical therapist come each time (the one day that wasn't possible was the day I described above). The agency honored our request as much as they were able and it made things much easier on Mom.

When we switched to hospice care, I made the same request and, after a few fumbles on the part of the hospice agency, during the most critical time before Mom's death, I was able to get the home health nurse who was temporarily doing hospice nursing to commit to being Mom's hospice nurse for the remainder of her life. That, frankly, by that point, made things easier for me to handle, and that's just as critical for us when crises or dying are in play.

It's also important to keep everything in the physical environment where it's supposed to be. Even moving a chair from one place to another can totally throw our loved ones off. We'll have time, if we're so inclined, to rearrange furniture and move things around as much as we want when our loved ones are gone, but while they're alive is not the time to do that.

One of the environmental disruptions that we may not think about, but need to eliminate, is rushing around, being "busy." The more we do this and the more people involved at the same time, the more disorienting it will be for our loved ones with dementias and Alzheimer's Disease. And this will trigger an avoidable mood swing.

The quieter and more evenly-paced we keep the physical environment for our loved ones, the less likely it will be that they will experience a lot of mood swings. The more chaotic, more frenzied, more loud we allow the physical environment for our loved ones with dementias and Alzheimer's Disease to get, the more likely it will be that mood swings will be a frequent fixture in our loved ones lives.

One other area in the physical environment that we should ensure is in place, as much as we're able, is having an established daily routine. This includes ensuring that meals are served at the same time each day. It means doing things in the same order throughout the day so that we create an atmosphere of security and comfort and safety.

Fear is often the underlying culprit in environmentally-based mood swings because changes and uncertainty cause a disproportionate amount of panic and anxiety for our loved ones with dementias and Alzheimer's Disease. By understanding this, we have a lot of control over minimizing and eliminating the sources of fear.

2. Physiological changes

Being sick, being in pain, or having a health crisis can trigger sudden and dramatic mood swings in our loved ones with dementias and Alzheimer's Disease. Even something as relatively benign as a cold can bring on severe mood fluctuations.

We, therefore, need to be vigilantly attentive to possible physiological changes that may be affecting our loved ones' moods. It's important to provide proper care immediately to minimize or eliminate physiology as a trigger for mood swings.

For things like colds, lots of fluids, hot soups, and tender loving care are the best remedies we can provide for our loved ones.

If pain is the issue for our loved ones with dementia and Alzheimer's Disease, then we need to get our care team involved and try to identify the source and cause of the pain and treat it.

Health crises, such as strokes, heart attacks, gallbladder infections, and chronic congestive heart failure, most often require that our loved ones be hospitalized. Mood swings will get more pronounced with hospitalizations because our loved ones are not only sick, but their environmental routines are totally turned up down: unfamiliar place, unfamiliar people, unfamiliar routine.

I always stayed with Mom when she was hospitalized. I was the only familiar face and I didn't want her to be there alone without anything that was familiar. Additionally, it meant that I could help her out when nurses and CNAs were busy or unavailable, so she never had to worry about nobody being there for her.

This was especially critical at night when Mom had her hearing aids off and even if she rang the call bell for help, she couldn't hear the answer (and why nurses never came down to check is a mystery to me – but Mom had told me years back when she had been in the hospital a few times that the nurses at night never answered her) so the nurses assumed it was a mistake.

This is the best comfort we can give our loved ones when they are hospitalized. They'll get funky with us too (I'd have to take breaks and go outside and walk and breathe to get calmed down sometimes when Mom was on a roll), but we're the only safety and security they've got, so we owe it to them to be there.

One of the most common physiological causes of mood swings, especially in older people, is urinary tract infections (UTIs). Often, these occur because of dehydration (not drinking enough fluids) or from improper toileting that allows bacteria (specifically, E. coli) to get into the urinary tract. Proper hydration and antibiotics can quickly clear urinary tract infections up.

So it's important if we see a sudden increase in confusion, mood swings, and behavioral issues in our loved ones with dementias and Alzheimer's Disease that we have them tested for a urinary tract infection, and if that's the cause, get them hydrated and on antibiotics as quickly as possible.

3. Perceptual changes

Perceptual changes – changes in hearing, comprehension, and vision – can also trigger mood swings. We gain context in life primarily through our senses: what we see, what we hear, what we taste, what we smell, what we feel by touch. Any situation in life – words and actions – where our senses are compromised or not intact change how we will perceive things.

For example, I am a better communicator in writing than I am verbally. I can be a decent communicator verbally, but not ad hoc. I have to have time to mentally process input and formulate my own thoughts to distill and crystalize a response. Most verbal exchanges don't build time into them, so I usually just opt for silence, since that's safe for me.

If I am involved in verbal communication, I prefer it to be one-on-one and face-to-face (Skype works as well, if not better, for me than in person because it's gives me a little breathing room) because I read facial expressions and body language to get context and to be able to perceive correctly.

Therefore, I absolutely hate to talk on the phone. I have none of the perceptual cues that I heavily depend on to communicate verbally and it greatly hinders my ability to be able to communicate even halfway decently in that environment.

In our loved ones with dementias and Alzheimer's Disease, all of their senses become skewed, so they begin responding to a skewed input. Comprehension and the ability to distinguish tone and nuance also decline, so everything that would give them the real context of words and actions to them and around them no longer works properly.

Fear is one factor that ensues. The other is confusion. These combined can create mood swings in our loved ones that are sudden and dramatic.

These are not insurmountable to handle, but they require us to slow down, be patient, be calm, and be reassuring.

It's imperative to make sure our loved ones understand, as well as they are able, what's going on around them. In essence, we become their senses and we help them with contexts they are no longer able to perceive.

This requires us to spend time explaining, re-explaining, and repeating ourselves as often as our loved ones need us to do it. That requires us to be patient. From experience, I can tell you that our loved ones may miss every loving gesture we show them, but they will catch and recognize (and react to) one exasperated sigh in a heartbeat.

I know it can be hard to answer the same questions and to make the same reassuring statements over and over. But I'll ask you – which is what I did and it made a world of difference in my patience with Mom – to put yourself in your little kid shoes with your parents and wear those again for a while.

How many times did you ask, on a trip, "Are we there yet?" How many times did you ask them the same things over and over? How many times did they have to reassure you about something new (and, therefore, scary) or something you were afraid of?

Yes, I know they got exasperated sometimes. Remember how that made you feel? But most of the time, they took us in their arms or held our hands and repeated the same answers and same assurances over and over and over, no matter how many times we needed to hear them.

We're completing the circle of life for them that they began with us. Notice what I said about touch. One of the most effective ways to calm our loved ones with dementias and Alzheimer's Disease is by touch: holding hands, putting an arm around their shoulders, embracing them in hugs, kissing them on the cheek. And never forget to say "I love you."

4. Neurological changes

   As damage to the brain progresses in dementias and Alzheimer's Disease, the areas of the brain that control mood and behavior are affected and this can be a trigger for mood swings as well.

   Vascular dementia is one type of dementia where extreme and abrupt mood swings are par for the course. Because vascular dementia is characterized by step-wise sudden and steep neurological declines, mood swings are much more in-your-face on a daily basis. If hadn't read about the chemistry behind Robert Louis Stevenson's *Dr. Jekyll and Mr. Hyde,* I would have pegged Dr. Jekyll as either schizophrenic or suffering from vascular dementia.

But other mood swings, such as uncontrollable rage, deepening depression (often as a result of our loved ones realizing they are losing themselves) and abject apathy are very common as neurological changes progress.

It's important to remember that the culprits for these are usually sadness, fear, and anxiety. A good anti-depressant and anti-anxiety medication (neither has to be a high dose) can often stabilize moods enough so that moods swings are less common and when they do occur - and they will - they are not as extreme.

Our responses to the neurological changes and resulting mood swings in our loved ones with dementias and Alzheimer's Disease can also be a big factor in their severity and duration.

Sometimes the best thing we can do is to remove ourselves from the line of fire. Because this is neurological damage, there is often nothing tangibly we can do for our loved ones to fix it, to persuade them, to change them from whatever state they're in emotionally. In fact, commonly, the more we try to do to intervene, the worse it gets.

However, we are responsible for not being the cause of further escalation, and sometimes just being in the same room with our loved ones is enough to cause that escalation. I can't explain it. And neither can anyone else. It's, as Spock from *Star Trek* would say, illogical.

But it happens. And when it does, it means we need to recognize when it's all bigger than us and walk away for a short period of time.

Our absence, even for a few minutes, will often be all that's need for our loved ones to get calmed down (not always, though – it may be several days that these mood swings persist and then it's a matter of going to separate corners when our loved ones don't need our help with something).

The intriguing thing is that most of the time it's like a switch that gets suddenly turned on and suddenly turned off. The problem is that neither we nor our loved ones with dementias and Alzheimer's Disease know when that switch is going to be activated and which position it will be in when it does.

If we don't need to remove ourselves from the line of fire, then it's imperative that we sit down with our loved ones and we listen, comfort, and reassure them.

Listening is the key here. Our loved ones know something's wrong and sometimes they just need the sympathetic ears of someone who loves them and will take the time to listen. That's our job.

Listening also can be beneficial because our loved ones with dementias and Alzheimer's Disease will have embedded somewhere in their conversations what's causing them to be afraid, to be sad, to be angry. And those are the things that we need to help them with, comfort them in, and reassure them about.

And, as always, a hug and kiss can go a long way in easing fears, sadness, and anger, even if it's the last thing we feel at that moment (love never dies, but it can be difficult when we've been on the receiving end of a mood).

Chapter 7: "Don't Know If It's Day Or Night"

Changes and disruptions in sleep are the next step in the journey our loved ones go through with dementias and Azheimer's Disease. Included in this step is a phenomenon called *sundowning*, which we'll explain the logic and science behind.

But first we need to talk about the science of sleep. All humans have a 24-hour internal clock that is known as our circadian clock (the term *circadian rhythm* refers to any biological process that completes a 24-hour cycle).

This clock, shown below, is a complex and coordinated system of neurology, hormones, environmental factors, and routines that are established from the time we are born.

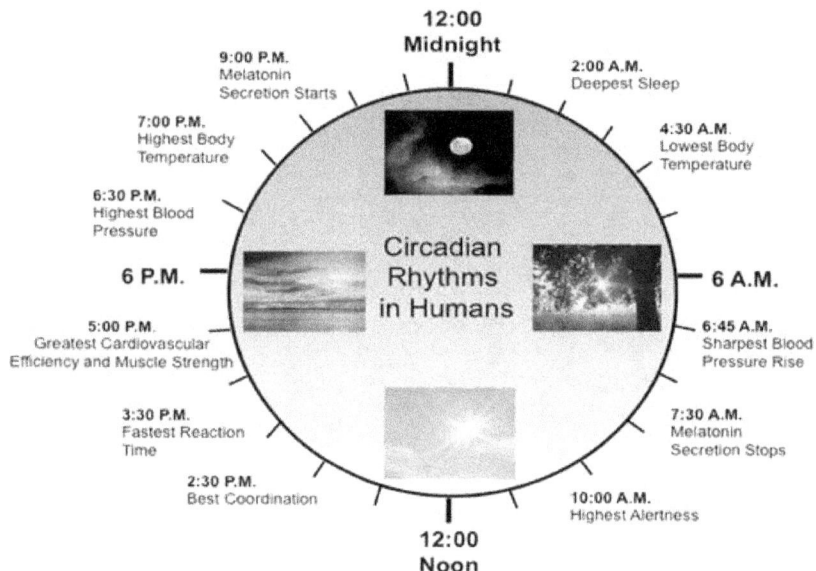

Everyone's circadian clock is unique, but each follows the general pattern shown above. In fact, the clock shown above is the ideal and the circadian clock that humans basically followed until the Industrial Revolution took place in the late 18th and early 19th centuries.

Since the full transition into the Industrial Revolution, human life and the adherence to this natural circadian clock has been altered and challenged because one of the side-effects of the Industrial Revolution was the development of artificial lighting (gas in the 19th century and electricity in the 20th century), which enabled lighting to be available 24 hours a day.

This was the byproduct of greed that served the captains of industry well (instead of limiting work hours to daylight hours only, artificial lighting enabled factories, foundries, mining operations, etc. to operate on a 24/7 schedule), but the human race definitely got the short end of the stick here.

Because the body is designed genetically, neurologically, hormonally, and environmentally to function in sync with the 24-hour circadian clock shown above, disrupted sleep and sleep deprivation has a chaotic effect on the body, even in otherwise-healthy people.

Time and again, science and medicine have shown a significant increase in accidents and serious injuries among shift workers who work at night. This includes not only production workers, but also professionals such as medical personnel. There is also a considerable amount of evidence that shows night shift workers are much likely to be injured or killed in driving accidents because they have a higher incidence of falling asleep behind the wheel going to and from work.

The most disruptive shift to the human body is the graveyard shift (usually 11 pm to 7 am). By the time these workers start their shift, the body is fully prepared (the hormone melatonin relaxes the body and mind for sleep beginning around 9 pm) to sleep. Forcing the body to do the complete opposite of what is it naturally designed to do is often counterproductive and very destructive to human health.

Even worse, at the time when these workers are getting off work, another hormone, cortisol, which "wakes" the body up is in full production, making sleep difficult, if not impossible, until much later in the day, and even the sleep then is not quantitative or qualitative. Sleep deprivation is the norm for these workers.

So seeing how disrupted sleep and sleep deprivation affects healthy people, it's not hard to see how exacerbated the effect of these sleep disturbances are on our loved ones with dementias and Alzheimer's Disease.

As people age, they tend to produce less melatonin, the hormone that prepares the body for sleep. This alone can lead to a lack of quality sleep and less sleep for older people. It is also not uncommon for older folks to take a few naps during the day – mainly because they're tired from not getting good and enough sleep at night – which makes being sleepy during normal sleeping hours less of a likelihood.

With our loved ones with dementias and Alzheimer's Disease, there are other complicating factors thrown on top of this. One is the decreasing ability to know what time it is, either by a clock or by the amount of natural light.

The two periods of the day that seem to be particularly difficult for them to distinguish between are dawn and dusk. Even healthy people on occasion can have the same difficulty.

I can think of a few times when I was so tired that I couldn't wait until bedtime to sleep and I took a power nap after work (usually after working almost around the clock with maybe two or three hours total sleep from Saturday night into the wee hours of Monday morning doing IT systems work that could be done only when nobody else was in the office, then having to be back in the office at 8 o'clock Monday morning and work all day) and when I woke up I was disoriented because I couldn't tell what time of the day it was. I would immediately panic thinking that I'd overslept and I was late getting up to go to work.

After I was awake for a few minutes, I was able to orient myself by external evidence to realize that it was dusk and not dawn.

However, our loved ones with dementia and Alzheimer's Disease don't have that same ability to cue themselves to the right time using external cues, so these are much more difficult times of day for them to distinguish.

In general, though, because of neurological changes causes by dementias and Alzheimer's Disease, our loved ones often lose the connection between the amount of light and wakefulness (the more light, the more awake, while the less light, the less awake), and it's not unusual for them to go to bed for the evening at strange times.

I remember my mom, one day in particular, being in her pajamas in bed for the night at 5 p.m. She will still living independently then, and I'd come in to wait with her for another sister to come in from out of town and we were going to take Mom to dinner.

I was surprised, but I also knew that by then Mom was up during the night, awake and walking, so I figured she was just tired and probably needed the sleep. Of course, when I woke her up she was understandably disoriented for a little while. I've often wondered if some of those middle-of-the-night walks were because Mom thought it was time to get up for the day.

One of the ways we can help with this problem is to ensure that there is a lot of available light during the day and then, as evening and bedtime draw near, dim the available light to orient our loved ones to daytime and nighttime. At night, however, it's a good idea to have a night light on, mostly for getting to the bathroom safely during the night, but also to ease night fears, especially with hallucinations and visuoperceptual problems, which are common in our loved ones with dementias and Alzheimer's Disease.

Another way that we can help our loved ones with better time orientation is to get a 24-hour digital clock, since we know that analog time is harder for them to process and because analog clocks don't indicate the time of day, even if our loved ones with dementias and Alzheimer's Disease can read them.

To illustrate the difference, this is a typical analog wall clock:

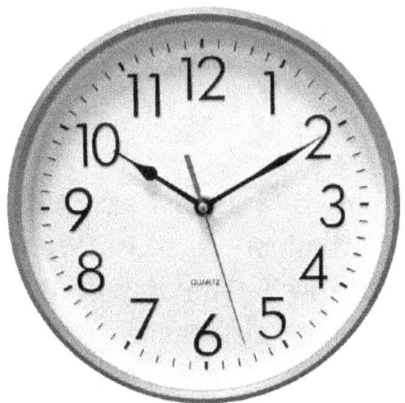

Even though the background is plain, the numbers are large and the long and short hands are pointed and distinct (useful for all older people), the only thing this clock can tell our loved ones is that it is 10:10. Without visual cues and/or knowledge, such as bright sunlight or darkness, this clock doesn't give any orientation about day or night.

On the other hand, a 24-hour digital clock gives our loved ones with dementias and Alzheimer's Disease much more information. I had a La Crosse Technology clock for my mom because it was easy to read and had comprehensive, uncluttered information, so that's the clock I'm showing here:

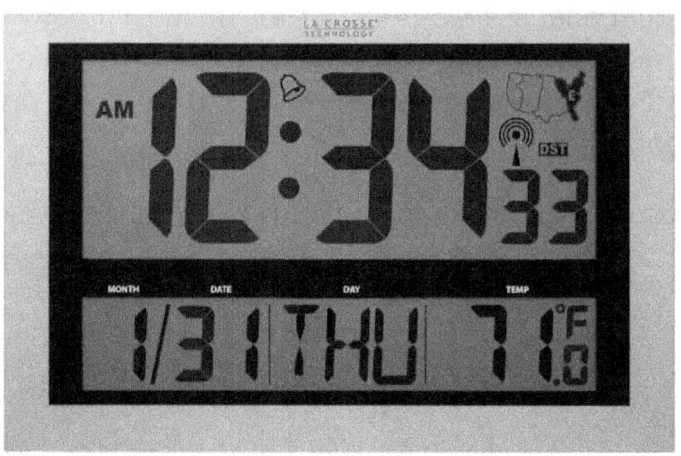

Note that everything is large and easy to read. While the time is displayed prominently, so is AM and PM. The day of the week is listed as well. The only thing that I would have liked to have seen done differently is to have the month abbreviation (in this case, Jan) spelled out instead of the number of the month, but I was never able to find a clock that didn't have this month/date format.

Since a decrease in production of the hormone melatonin is also a factor in sleep disturbances and sleep deprivation in a lot of older people, and not just our loved ones with dementias and Alzheimer's Disease, compensating for that decrease is something that needs to be addressed.

Often medical personnel will push for a prescription sleep medications like Ambien® (generic form is zolpidem) or Lunesta® to treat sleep disturbances in our loved ones. We have the right – and should – refuse these kinds of medications because of the side effects and safety risks associated with them.

I am adamantly opposed to using them anywhere in the elderly population because of their rapid effect and the subsequent fall risk associated with not being able to move quickly enough to safely lie down before the medication starts working.

I personally know of an elderly lady in her late 80's, who was sharp as a tack, had no health problems, and was living independently who was prescribed Ambien by her doctor. One night when the medication took effect this lady was between the bathroom and her bedroom. She fell hard, broke both hips, and never walked again. The lady spent the last few years of her life bedbound in a nursing home.

However, in our loved ones with dementias and Alzheimer's Disease, using prescription sleep medications can have even more profound and dangerous effects.

One of those is increased confusion. Most of these medications contain chemical combinations that are designed to adjust brain chemistry in a normally-functioning brain to induce sleep.

However, because dementias and Alzheimer's Disease create abnormally-functioning brains, brain chemistry is also significantly affected. Therefore, the targets of these prescription sleep medications are either severely impaired or not even present all the time. Therefore, whatever brain chemistry is present gets affected and the result is greater confusion both during the day and at night.

Another effect is excessive grogginess during the day. Because these medications can't be utilized and metabolized correctly by our loved ones with dementias and Alzheimer's Disease, they tend to have a longer half-life in the body and the effects can continue even through daytime hours, acting almost like a sedative and our loved ones have no quality awake time.

Some medications like Ambien® have the effect of getting a person to sleep, but not keeping them asleep. However, a person awakening with Ambien in his or her system is essentially sleepwalking. There have been several well-publicized instances of that with this medication over the years.

Because of the increased tendency to wander (which we'll discuss in the next chapter), especially at night, in our loved ones with dementias and Alzheimer's Disease, the possibility of sleepwalking can be even more dangerous and even fatal.

The best, safest, and most natural way that we can ensure our loved ones get as much quality sleep as they can is to supplement the decreased level of melatonin that occurs with aging. Melatonin can be purchased over-the-counter at drug stores and big-box retailers like WalMart and Target.

Although up to 12 mg of melatonin supplementation a day is considered safe, don't start at this level. Remember the goal: a good night's sleep. Therefore, I recommend starting with the lowest dosage (1 mg), adjusting upward until our loved ones with dementias and Alzheimer's Disease are consistently sleeping well at night. Generally, that dosage should be effective through the end of the disease process.

My mom started with 3 mg of melatonin per day – always give this with any other bedtime medications – recommended by her primary care physician. Eventually, we increased the dosage to 5 mg per day and that was an effective dose for her to get a good night's sleep (when her R.E.M. sleep disorder associated with Lewy Body dementia worsened from time to time, I increased her melatonin dosage to 7 mg per day for the duration, which seemed to help, then decreased it back to 5 mg per day when those particular symptoms subsided).

The good news is that melatonin has none of the side effects – increased confusion, grogginess, etc. – that prescription sleep medications can cause.

However, it's important to remember to let members of our loved ones' care teams know, if we start the melatonin on our own, that we've added it and what the dosage is.

One more note related to prescription sleep medications and hospital admissions, which are often on the as-needed list of medications, especially at night when agitation and sleep disturbances can be worst, is that we must advocate for our loved ones as to whether any medication like this can be administered, and, if so, at what dosage, and under what circumstances.

Hospitals tend to rely on Haldol (which is specifically contraindicated for elderly patients with dementia), Ativan, Restoril, and Resperdal for sleep issues, and they also tend to give relatively high doses. None of these drugs is specifically formulated for sleep – they are in the anti-anxiety and anti-psychosis classes of drugs.

These prescription medications all tend to produce very negative side effects in our loved ones, even in low dosages.

However, in my experience with the two times that Mom had Ativan in the hospital (I refused to let them give it to her anymore after that) is that the night staff tended to administer higher and more frequent dosages basically because it made things easier and quieter for them.

But the repercussions were severe and dangerous-to-potentially-fatal in at least one instance.

Generally, by this step of the progression of dementias and Alzheimer's Disease, our loved ones will already have anti-anxiety medication on board as part of their daily medications. And if our loved ones are already taking a melatonin supplement, that combined with the anti-anxiety medication they normally take should be all they need at night to get some sleep – hospitals are not conducive to a good night's sleep for anyone – during the night.

There is another important aspect of the disrupted 24-hour circadian clock that our loved ones with dementias and

Alzheimer's Disease experience and that is the phenomenon known as *sundowning*. The name of this unusual and repetitive daily occurrence comes from the fact that it typically occurs in the hours on either side of the sun setting.

What it looks like is speech and behavior repetition, increased agitation, restlessness, pacing, and perhaps even some aggravation and aggressiveness in our loved ones. Even if our loved ones have been calm and fairly composed all day, this time of day will suddenly bring on a flurry of activity and it may seem impossible to get our loved ones settled back down.

There are several probable explanations for sundowning.

One explanation is that by this time of day, the energy levels of our loved ones are depleted, which can cause increased anxiety and stress. Additionally, lessening light seems to trigger more distress and anxiousness as well (this is, in some ways, tied to visuoperceptual problems as well).

Another explanation is that this time of day releases a long-term memory trigger that tells our loved ones they need to be up and busy doing something. This makes sense because when our loved ones with dementias and Alzheimer's Disease were healthy and active, this time of day was usually busiest for them. They were coming home from work to their families and household activities, including activities like getting kids to do homework, doing laundry, cleaning the house, feeding pets, getting dinner ready, and perhaps doing yard work or working in vegetable or flower gardens during the spring and summer months.

A third explanation goes hand-in-hand with the second explanation: this is still often the busiest and most multitasking time of day for us as caregivers and for our families. As our loved ones watch our households in varied and somewhat-frenzied activities, while they may just be sitting somewhere because they are tired, it seems that they both get "worked up" by all the activity and the anxiety and stress of everything going on around them brings out the sundowning behaviors.

While sundowning occurs typically only through mid-stage (what we're discussing) dementias and Alzheimer's Disease, it can be very difficult to deal with.

There are some very easy and practical ways to help alleviate this anxiety and stress in our loved ones.

The easiest is to maintain a daily routine that doesn't deviate (this may mean that we keep activities calmed down during the hours around sunset by doing as much of our "busy" work at other times during the day or after our loved ones have gone to bed), so our loved ones with dementias and Alzheimer's Disease feel safe and comfortable.

Another very practical way is to, as we're able, involve our loved ones in activities like getting dinner ready so that they can both be with us and participate with us, which will also give them something to do to feel productive and will also reassure them that we're there and they are safe.

The worst possible thing we can do is to respond to our loved ones with dementias and Alzheimer's Disease who are sundowning with frustration, anger, screaming, yelling, and exasperation. This will only escalate their behavior and it will not turn out well for anybody.

It's important, once again, for us to remember that our loved ones with dementias and Alzheimer's Disease are not behaving like this intentionally or on purpose.

We can count to 10 and take a bunch of deep breaths, if we need to, but we have to stay calm and be comforting and reassuring with our loved ones.

We're the only ones capable of managing the situation successfully, so the responsibility is on us to do everything in our power to let our loved ones with dementias and Alzheimer's Disease know that everything's fine, they're safe, we're there, and we're going to be there and make sure they're okay.

A little gentleness and a little kindness and a lot of love will go a long way in helping our loved ones maneuver well through this step of dementias and Alzheimer's Disease.

Chapter 8: "Can't Find My Way Home"

Wandering is the next step of the journey our loved ones with dementias and Alzheimer's Disease go through. Wandering can be characterized by endless walking within the safety of a house or facility, but more often it is characterized by going outside and either walking or driving (if our loved ones are still driving) aimlessly until our loved ones are lost and either can't or don't know they need to or how to come back.

There are many stories of elderly people with dementias and Alzheimer's Disease who were wandering on foot or in a vehicle who died before they could be located. These people have been hit by vehicles while walking in the middle of the street, walked into woods and gotten lost, or have driven vehicles off the road over embankments or into bodies of water.

Often, the impulsive nature of wandering – a sudden need to be stimulated or being on a mission to go somewhere or find something – leads our loved ones with dementias and Alzheimer's Disease to just pick up and go, often without adequate clothing in cold weather, and often in the middle of the night.

Wandering may be tied to visual hallucinations as well, especially if the visual hallucination is of a loved one. When that person leaves, our loved ones may want to follow and go with them.

However, the main impetus of wandering seems to be rooted in the desire to *go home*. Our loved ones with dementias and Alzheimer's Disease begin talking frequently about wanting to go home – even if they're in a home they've lived in for many years – and wanting to find loved ones, many of whom have been dead for years.

It's important to understand the context of where our loved ones with dementias and Alzheimer's Disease are neurologically and memory-wise. While dementias and Alzheimer's Disease affect short-term memory and inhibit new memories from being formed, long-term memories are and stay, for most of the duration, intact. And those long-term memories are where our loved ones begin spending a lot of time.

Therefore, *home*, for our loved ones is most often their childhood or early adulthood homes, and those homes and the people who were there are what our loved ones are looking for and where they want to go.

I remember my mom telling us kids a story about her paternal grandmother, who was in her 80's and "senile." Mom's grandmother was living with her daughter and her family on the family farm in the family home in a little town in rural northeast Tennessee. Day after day Mom's grandmother, accompanied by her daughter's sons who were sent with Grandma to make sure she was safe and to get her back home when she was tired, walked for hours up and down the dirt roads around the farm looking for the younger version of her daughter.

I remember another story about a lady who lived in the retirement community where Mom lived. She left on foot one night and when the police found her she was eight miles away walking down a four-lane road toward the home she and her late husband had owned in another town.

Mom did her own wandering at night when she was at the retirement community. I know of the one instance when she went to the military recruiting station a block or so away – it faced one of the busiest roads where we lived – to ask them (because I believe she thought they were the police) to arrest me and ended up being transported to the hospital for evaluation.

How many more times Mom wandered at night and where she went, I don't know. But I do know that thinking about it makes me both anxious and thankful that she never got lost, hurt, or killed if she did (I assume she did, but it's probably best that I don't know for sure).

But with Mom's wandering came the desire to go home. Home for her was the same house that her grandmother had wandered around all those years ago looking for the younger version of her daughter. I would drive Mom out to the house frequently, because that's where she wanted to go, but it suddenly, on Memorial Day 2010, became, to Mom, *Grandpa's house*.

All the years up until then, the house had always been Mom's aunt's house. The day it became *Grandpa's house*, I knew something had changed with Mom. She loved her grandfather dearly. He died in that house when Mom was five years old, and from that point on the loving, safe childhood Mom had known unraveled quickly, disappearing completely within 18 months of her grandfather's death.

Going home for Mom, then, was going back to the years before her grandfather died and to the home they shared together.

Although wandering can be a scary aspect of dementias and Alzheimer's Disease, it can be managed quite successfully and quite easily.

Since wandering can be tied to a lack of stimulation (kids tend to do the same thing when they're bored or can't focus – one of my sisters wandered around her first-grade classroom so often that it became the subject of several parent-teacher conferences and led to her being fitted with her first pair of glasses because her bad eyesight was the reason she couldn't focus), one of the ways that it can be managed is to keep our loved ones with dementias and Alzheimer's Disease busy and active during the day with things that interest them and that they are able to successfully do. This will help with sleep, but it will also keep their minds occupied and them busy and it will give them a sense of being productive and accomplishing things.

One of the things that Mom and I did together almost on a daily basis until she wasn't able to anymore was work on 300-piece large-piece jigsaw puzzles.

We listened to music a lot. Research has shown that music is incredibly therapeutic for our loved ones with dementias and Alzheimer's Disease and can activate areas of the brain that are otherwise inaccessible and stimulate memories and conversation. I created several playlists on Spotify (a customizable internet jukebox) for Mom that included her favorite artists and the different kinds of music she liked and I'd put them on shuffle so we'd have a random variety each time I played the lists.

We'd do some kind of physical activity every day, including taking walks outside together when the weather was nice, as much as much as Mom was able to physically handle, bouncing a ball back and forth in the kitchen, pedaling on a little mini-bicycle, and doing strengthening and core exercises that her physical therapist would give us on each visit.

We also did household chores together, with me doing the things that required agility and good processing skills and Mom doing the things that she could do sitting or standing beside me with me ensuring that she didn't fall.

On a daily basis, we'd sit and read books together, with Mom and me taking turns reading until she was no longer able to read out loud, and then I would read to her. Along the way, we would talk about what we were reading.

Sometimes, I'd pull out coloring books and crayons and we'd sit at the kitchen table and color with the goal of being the most creative and innovative in choosing colors for our pictures. Mom always got that honor because she always had a much livelier imagination than I did.

When it was safe and she could sit at the table, Mom would help me with cooking. I'd often let her help make salads by tearing up the lettuce while I chopped vegetables, then I'd put them in bowls and let her put them on each salad. When I baked cookies or crackers, I'd make the dough and Mom would spoon it out onto the baking sheets. After they cooled, Mom would put them in airtight storage containers.

One of the games that Mom and I played a lot until the last few months of her life was checkers. She amazingly had a fair amount of strategic ability left and it was rare that she didn't beat me. I didn't hold back and let her win either. She beat me fair and square on her own ability. Of course, I was happy that she could do that and would make a really big deal out of her winning.

These are just a few ideas for us to take and build on. There are many things that our loved ones with dementias and Alzheimer's Disease can do to help out, to be productive, and to be mentally stimulated.

But as it is with children when they first begin learning to do things and helping with chores, including our loved ones in these activities will require time (they will be slower and can often process the activity one step at a time with repetition), patience, and attention.

One thing I learned to accept was that any effort was good enough. As Mom declined neurologically, even though she continued to help me with chores like folding laundry and doing prep work for meals, her ability to do them well and neatly declined as well. I tend to be a little obsessive-compulsive about neatness and doing things just so and a certain way, and I had to let go of that with Mom and realize that her wanting to help me and being able to help me was more important than things being done well or neatly.

There are also some easy environmental solutions to prohibit wandering outside. One of the simplest uses the visuoperceptual problem of *visual cliffs,* which are common among our loved ones with dementias and Alzheimer's disease.

Visual cliffs are visual distortions characterized by sudden stops from our loved ones at door thresholds and on walking surfaces where there are marked changes in color and consistency (such as going from a wood floor to a tile floor or from carpet to a tiled floor). The causes of the sudden stops are abnormal depth perception and the fear of falling.

By putting something as simple as 2" black tape across the bottom of all exterior doors, we can create a visual cliff that can prevent our loved ones with dementias and Alzheimer's Disease from opening the doors and going outside.

Since nighttime wandering is a big concern, we can invest in fairly inexpensive door alarms (if our homes have a security system already, then setting it at night will do the trick) that go off if exterior doors are open. There are also inexpensive bed and chair alarms that we can place under our loved ones while they are sitting or sleeping (under their bottoms is best). Any movement to get up, which involves weight shifting of their bottoms, will make the alarms go off.

Additionally, if our loved ones with dementias and Alzheimer's Disease are sleeping in separate rooms from our rooms, investing in a baby monitor (preferably with video) is an excellent idea.

The bottom line is that although wandering can be scary, it doesn't have to be and there are a lot of creative ways that we can minimize or eliminate it.

Chapter 9: "I Keep On Fallin'"

While many of our loved ones with dementias and Alzheimer's Disease are in good shape physically when these diseases begin to manifest themselves, they eventually reach this step of the journey where there is a great risk of falling. Attached to this risk is the possibility of broken bones - especially hips, which may be so badly damaged that our loved ones become confined to wheelchairs or bed for the rest of their lives - and head injuries, which can be fatal.

The reasons that our loved ones are increasingly susceptible to falls are:

1. Gait changes

   Gait changes are common as dementias and Alzheimer's Disease progress in our loved ones. One of the most characteristic gait changes is *shuffling*. This is especially pronounced in our loved ones who have Lewy Body dementia and Parkinson's Disease, but it becomes a feature of all dementias and Alzheimer's Disease by this step of the journey.

   Shuffling is when our loved ones don't pick their feet up off the floor to take steps, but instead slide them across the floor to move forward. One of the inherent dangers in this is catching the front part of shoes on the floor - especially carpet - and falling forward.

Shuffling can be both a result of neurological impairment – not remembering how to take normal steps to walk – and muscle weakness from lack of use.

The most important thing we can do for our loved ones with dementias and Alzheimer's Disease to help minimize shuffling is to have a physical therapist on our care teams to help regain muscle strength and work on gait normalization. Additionally, if possible, we should be helping our loved ones maintain muscle strength and walk with them daily encouraging them, both by example and by instruction, to use a normal stepping gait to walk.

Additionally, we should ensure that our loved ones with dementias and Alzheimer's Disease have a walker when they are walking (we'll discuss the type of walkers available and their appropriateness during the progression of these diseases a little later in this chapter).

We also need to be with our loved ones when every time they are up and walking. And one of the most helpful things that we should have to help our loved ones with dementias and Alzheimer's Disease is a gait belt.

A gait belt is not only used for hanging on to our loved ones while they're walking, but is critical for helping them to stand and sit down as dementias and Alzheimer's Disease progress and they have more difficulty standing and sitting. Gait belts will also help in lifting our loved ones who, because of muscle weakness and/or neurological impairment, are essentially "dead weight" because they're unable to assist us in standing, especially.

There are many kinds of gait belts on the market. From my experience using them, I would recommend one with a quick-release snap-together buckle with handles on the sides (lifting to stand and guiding back into a sitting position) and the back (holding to prevent falls while walking). The handles give you the leverage that you won't find on the standard gait belts that most medical facilities and physical therapists use.

The Posey Six-Handle Gait Belt (http://www.wrightstuff.biz/posixhagabe.html) is my recommendation for a good gait belt. It looks like this:

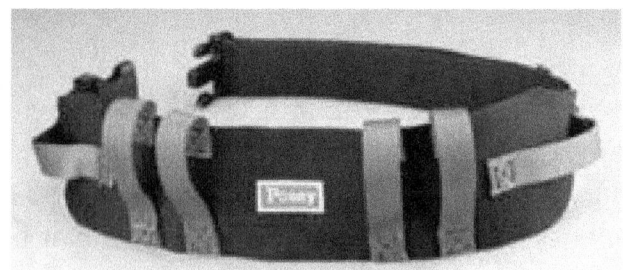

2. Balance problems

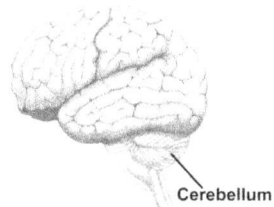

Cerebellum

The cerebellum is responsible for balance and physical coordination. When it is damaged – and this is usually one of the first indications of vascular dementia – balance and coordination are significantly affected.

My mom started falling more frequently long before she was diagnosed with vascular dementia. She couldn't explain why she fell (she usually told me "the next thing I knew I was on the floor or on the ground"), but the falls increased over the years. Fortunately, other than some pretty nasty bruises on occasion, she escaped any serious injuries.

One thing that I was never able to explain was that when she was in the geriatric psychiatric hospital, she suddenly began turning around the opposite way that people normally turn around and she'd lose her balance. That continued the rest of her life and it was responsible for several falls.

Near the end of her life, Mom had almost no balance standing and I could not let her stand without me holding on to her for even a few seconds or she'd fall backwards. That was indicative of pretty extensive damage to her cerebellum.

3. Physical Weakness

The less muscles get used, the more they will atrophy and the weaker they will become. The leg muscles may atrophy to the point where they are not able to support the weight of the upper body and falls will be more likely.

4. Visuoperceptual problems

Visuoperceptual problems such as the sudden stops that accompany visual cliffs are also a factor in our loved ones being more prone to falling. The problem is that when the body is in a forward motion and that motion is suddenly stopped, the upper half of the body is still going forward, and the weight of the body will shift forward, resulting in a face-down fall.

5. Clutter

If our loved ones with dementias and Alzheimer's Disease have a lot of clutter to try to walk around, falls are more likely to occur. It is important for us to make sure that are walking areas are clear and there are no obstacles to have to sidestep, walk around, or walk over.

6. Fatigue

   Just as is true with little kids, our loved ones with dementias and Alzheimer's Disease will be more apt to fall when they are physically tired. With neurological impairment, the brain, even at the greatest point of wakefulness, is not functioning well. With fatigue, the lack of functioning gets more pronounced and falls are more likely.

   The remedy for this is that we need to be aware when our loved ones are getting physically tired and we need to ensure that they are sitting or lying down before they're completely worn out so that no falls and injuries can occur.

7. Medication side effects

   Medications can often have side effects like dizziness, which can cause our loved ones with dementias and Alzheimer's Disease to be more likely to fall.

   If we notice after medications are changed or added that the risk of falling is greater, it is imperative that we, with our loved ones, consult with our care teams to address eliminating the medication or changing to a similar medication with less side effects.

Preventing falls in our loved ones with dementias and Alzheimer's Disease requires us to be attentive and available at all times. That means that each time they get up and walk, we need to be right behind them, assisting them, and doing our best to ensure that they are safe while they are up and moving around.

My mom was a great fall risk toward the end of her life. Her balance was gone. I left her standing one day, holding on to her walker, for no more than 10 seconds, because I needed to get something before she sat down in her recliner – I was two steps away from her – and she fell backwards in the hallway.

Ironically, there was one day about two weeks later (about a month before her death) when we were going to the funeral home because Mom wanted to be sure that everything was set for her funeral arrangements, that while I was trying to get ready upstairs, Mom kept getting up and walking around anxiously and didn't fall at all.

Of course, I was a nervous wreck because every time I heard her locks click off on the walker, I ran downstairs and tried to get Mom to sit down and wait for me to get dressed. I don't remember how many times I ended up doing that, but it was several, and I know I finally raised my voice the last time I asked her to sit down and wait for me to finish getting dressed, not because I was angry, but because I was terrified that she was really going to get hurt.

Once we got in the car, Mom calmed down. And by the time we got to the funeral home, Mom was really tired and I used a wheelchair to get her in and out of the funeral home.

After we left the funeral home, Mom wanted to go out to the graveyard where her family and my dad were buried and where she would be buried. Although Mom, with my assistance, was able to walk with her walker down the first row of graves where her family was buried, unlike every previous visit to the graveyard, she didn't talk about any of them or linger. I called out the names as we walked by and when we got to her dad's grave she nodded her head and said she was ready to go home.

One of other the ways that we can help prevent falls is by having our loved ones use a walker to assist them with walking. There are three basic types of walkers available – the first type is non-rolling and the other two types are rolling – shown below:

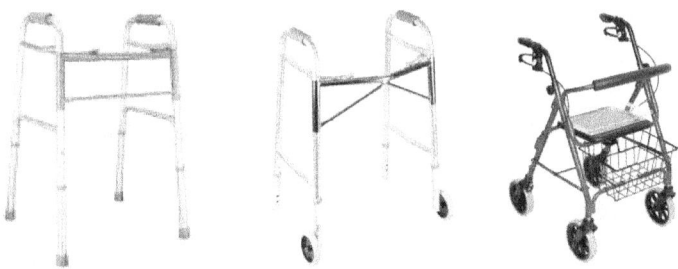

Each of these types of walkers can be useful through the progression of these diseases.

The rollator walker is a good walker for our loved ones with dementias and Alzheimer's Disease in the early stages of needing support while they are walking. It features wheels, which make moving at a normal pace natural and easier, and it has both a braking and a locking system.

Rollators are the most expensive type of walker (Medicare will pay for one walker, so if this is the first one our loved ones with dementias and Alzheimer's Disease get, Medicare will cover the cost) and they are not adjustable so our loved ones will need to be custom-fitted with one that matches their heights.

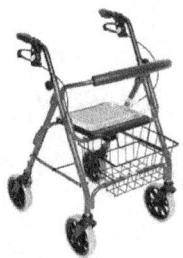

It's important to try to help our loved ones maintain an upright posture while using any walker - what often happens is that people using walkers tend to bend over and lean on them while walking and this is bad for the neck, shoulders, and back – but it's also important that the walker is set correctly for their heights.

One of the really nice – and smart - features of the rollator is the seat (buying a basket is usually extra, but it is a nice addition too). The seat can be used to transport things from one place to another, but it can also be used to provide a seat for our loved ones to sit on if they get tired while they are out walking around. The brakes should always be locked when using the rollator as a place to sit.

However, one of the rollator's disadvantages is that it is extremely lightweight and cannot be safely, unless we are holding it still, used to assist our loved ones with standing from a seated position. It will tip over and could cause serious injuries.

The other disadvantage of the rollator comes into play as our loved ones progress in the journey of dementias and Alzheimer's Disease. The wheels that make it move so easily can cause the rollator to get away from our loved ones quickly resulting in falls. Additionally, as these neurological diseases progress, the ability to use the safety features of the rollator - the brakes and the locks - will diminish and make its use risky.

The next type of walker has straight legs in the back and wheels on the front. This is what I consider an intermediate walker between the four-legged walker and the rollator. Because it has only two wheels, it will still move fairly easily in conjunction with walking, but it is easier to control and stop.

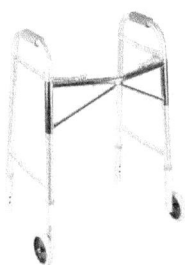

Notice that it is wider than the rollator. That extra width gives it a little more stability for our loved ones to go from a sitting to standing position easily, but we should still be there to hold the walker when our loved ones are standing.

One of the other features of this walker is that it's adjustable, and it can almost be customized to match the height of our loved ones.

The third type of walker has four straight legs. Like the two-wheeled walker, it is wide and it is adjustable. This walker is suitable for the later stages of dementias and Alzheimer's as well as for other health conditions that may make walking more cumbersome for our loved ones.

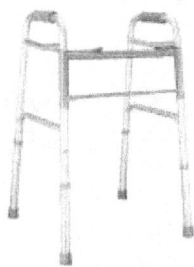

This walker slows the pace of walking considerably, because to walk with it, our loved ones have to pick it up, move it forward a little, then step into it, so to speak. At this stage, we are going to need to be with them every step of the way, so we will likely having to do coaching on how to use the walker and how to move forward.

Mom had a rollator walker almost until the end and she did well with it for the most part (I was never far away, and the last few months of her life, I walked right behind her, holding on to her, any time she was walking).

But Mom had a major heart attack a week and a half before she died and it did a lot of damage to her heart. Mom slept for the better part of two days after the heart attack, waking up for short periods of time three or four times.

Each time Mom woke up, we took a few steps together to the bedside commode, where she could toilet and I could help her get washed up and changed into clean clothes, but even those few steps were hard for her.

When her heart had recovered to the point that Mom was more alert and awake, she still could not walk very far and I realized that the rollator was no longer a safe option for her to use walking.

I had hospice deliver a four-legged walker (Medicare pays for this under hospice care). It took a few days after Mom's heart attack before she could walk very much or even to the bathroom, but this walker made that much easier for Mom when she was able to.

So while the risk of falls increases with the progression of dementias and Alzheimer's Disease, there are many things that we can do to recognize when falls are likely and prevent them – you will not prevent them all and they will tear up your heart when they happen – and keep our loved ones active and safe throughout these neurological diseases.

Chapter 10: "Time Reverse And Rewind"

The next step in the journey with our loved ones with dementias and Alzheimer's Disease can be difficult to comprehend and adjust to, since it usually appears randomly and unexpectedly. This step is where our loved ones seem to frequently go back in time in memories, in conversations, and in thinking and they often don't recognize us or know who we are.

I first read Katherine Anne Porter's *The Jilting of Granny Weatherall* in high school. It is the story of an 80-year-old woman who has dementia and/or Alzheimer's Disease. Neither of these names for neurological impairment existed, however, when Porter wrote this short story in 1930. Instead, elderly people were just "senile."

The story made a strong impression on me even as a teenager, even though I never had steady and intimate contact with elderly people (both my parents lost their parents when they were very young and, as only children who were much younger than their cousins, had no aunts and uncles except one on my mom's side left by the times we kids came along) and had never seen anything that looked like dementias and Alzheimer's Disease.

I found Granny Weatherall fascinating and I found the juxtaposition of where she was in her own mind versus what was actually going on around her intriguing.

If you have not read the story, you should.

You can find a PDF copy of it online at http://www.qcc.mass.edu/booth/255/files/Porter-Jilting.pdf.

Granny Weatherall, like our loved ones with dementias and Alzheimer's Disease, spends a lot of her time jumping from place to place in her past, occasionally – and seldom willingly or happily - coming back to the present, but often unaware of time and unable to recognize the daughter she lives with. While our loved ones may not be unhappy or unwilling to come back to the present, their transport most of the time to the past will very strongly resemble Granny Weatherall's.

In the last eight months of my mom's life, I thought of this story quite often when Mom would talk about the distant past like it was the recent past or present, when she would have hallucinations about a man and small children (it had to have been my dad and us kids when we were little) in the house with us, when she would ask me about my parents, if they were living, where they lived, and where I was attending college and what I was studying.

I will never forget the first time it happened. Mom and I had just finished dinner in late December 2011. We had been chatting at the table about things when, out of the blue, Mom asked me where my parents lived.

It shocked me, but unlike most of the time when something completely throws me off guard and I either can't respond or don't respond well, I didn't miss a beat and answered

Mom. She then asked me if my parents were still alive. I answered that too.

Then Mom asked me who my parents were. I told Mom that dad had died and I pointed at her and said, "You're my mom."

It was Mom's turn to be surprised. She asked, with a surprised look on her face, "I am?" I answered that she was.

In all of this, I really didn't understand why Mom was asking me what she was asking me. I knew something was amiss, but it wasn't until later that evening that I realized why Mom was asking me the questions that she was asking.

After I cleared off the table, Mom and I went into the living room to sit and work on a jigsaw puzzle. We talked in the present until Mom looked up at me and asked me where I was going to college. Suddenly I realized that Mom didn't know who I was. I gave her the name of the actual college I went to. Mom then asked me what I was studying. I gave her the major that I actually got my degree in.

We spent the rest of that evening vacillating between the present and the past and the unknown, and while it was disconcerting to me on one level, it was fascinating to me on another.

During the next eight months, we'd have these kinds of conversations from time to time.

The last week that Mom was alive, she didn't know me most of the time. I don't know that she actually knew where she was, even though we were at home, most of the time. I didn't realize this right away, but I understood eventually because of what Mom would say to me.

One of the most touching memories of that week was the first clue I had that Mom was not with me in the present. I'd gotten her into bed one night with some difficulty and, although she wasn't hurt at all, she was upset with me.

In the very early hours of the next morning, I bolted upright out of the chair I was sleeping in with a very painful cramp in my calf. I saw that Mom was awake too, but she wasn't trying to get up, but instead was watching me. I tried to walk the cramp out and it got worse and then I sat down in another chair and massaged my calf until the pain was bearable.

I then went over to Mom's bed and I hugged her and leaned down to ask in her good ear if she was okay and whether she needed anything. She pulled me close in a bear hug and said "I know I can't get out of here, but when you feel better, you leave as soon as you can. Promise me."

With tears streaming down my face, I told Mom that I loved her and I would. Mom was right. I needed to get out of this place, especially since all the reasons I had to be here – in fact, why I was here – are gone. I'm still trying to get out of this place, but it hasn't happened as quickly as I had thought or hoped.

Mom went back to sleep and I went back to the chair and dozed until morning. As we were eating breakfast the next morning, Mom looked around furtively and leaned over close to me and very conspiratorially said to me "I don't want *that woman* to hear me, but *that woman* is mean to me." It dawned on me that Mom was talking about the hard time I had getting her into bed the evening before. I told Mom that she didn't have anything to worry about and that *that woman* probably wasn't mean, but that I thought she just didn't know what she was doing.

Mom's relief was palpable when I told her this.

The rest of the week was similar with Mom drifting seamlessly from the present to the past and back. By Friday, Mom was talking about me in the third person. She desperately wanted me to be there with her, but she didn't realize that I already was.

On Saturday, Mom rallied and recognized me and was delighted to see me. She stayed in the present that day with my sister and me and it was a day filled with good conversations, laughter, and a lot of love.

By Sunday morning, even though Mom was still very much in the present and happy, I knew her kidneys had begun to shut down. At around 1:30 pm that afternoon, Mom's whole demeanor changed and she started complaining of chest pains. I gave her morphine as prescribed and she looked at my sister and me and said the last words of her life: "I guess they're going to throw me out now."

We both comforted Mom, and I took both her hands and reassured her that she was home, we loved her, and we weren't going to kick her out. She went to sleep, our hands clasped together, and died two days later without ever waking up again.

It wasn't until four months later that I realized that Mom's statement about being thrown out was an indication that she had gone back to her distant past that Sunday afternoon: the only thing Mom was ever "thrown out" (her words every time she talked about it) of was nursing school in the early 1950's because of her hearing loss.

The is the most critical thing that we can do with our loved ones who have dementias and Alzheimer's Disease is always tell the truth. In all my answers to Mom, I was always truthful with her. I never made anything up and I never lied about anything.

Honesty is part of integrity and trust and it is part of our character. Once we compromise that, then we destroy trust and we destroy integrity and we destroy our character. That shouldn't be acceptable to any of us. After all, do we want people lying to us and making things up?

One of the tenets that a lot of the books, blogs, and websites that discuss dementias and Alzheimer's Disease promote is the telling of "fiblets." These are lies, no matter how innocuous this word may sound. If we do this, we're being dishonest and we are untrustworthy.

The reason these sources recommend telling "fiblets" is ostensibly to calm our loved ones down when they're in the past or don't recognize us, but the reality is that these lies are told with the assumption that they will make our lives easier in the short-term.

The problem is that lies don't make anything easier. And resorting to lying really says a lot about how unwilling we are to take the time, to listen, to meet our loved ones where they are, and really communicate with them in a way that is gentle, calming, and honest.

I always met Mom where she was and I listened a lot. I never tried to get her back to the present nor did I get upset because she was back in time trying to work things out.

I listened for the most part, asking her questions when I could tell that she was trying to make peace with something in her past, and answering her honestly when she asked me questions. I learned a lot that way.

We can all learn a lot that we may not know by handling this step of the journey of dementias and Alzheimer's Disease with patience, with gentleness, with listening, and with truthfulness.

Chapter 11: "I'm Just A Little Unwell"

As our loved ones progress through dementias and Alzheimer's Disease, medical care will become a more central and ever-present part of the journey. It's important that we understand this and are prepared in every way possible to become team leaders and advocates for our loved ones to ensure that they receive the right care, the best care, and, as much as they are able, are actively involved in medical discussions, decisions, and care.

At this step of the journey, it is too late to determine finite boundaries of care and to create legal documents designating powers of attorney, living wills, and Do Not Resuscitate (DNR) orders because our loved ones are not considered competent to make these kinds of decisions.

So it is imperative that these decisions and documents are discussed, if not well in advance of the initial signs of dementias and Alzheimer's Disease, at least in the earliest stages, when our loved ones can decide what they want and convey and formalize those wishes.

In fact, we all should do this, no matter where we are in life. We should have wills, living wills, DNR's (if that's what we want). We should talk to the people that we designated to ensure our wishes are fulfilled and let them know that they are responsible and what we want and don't want.

In addition, someone should have all our financial, insurance, and digital (online access to bank accounts, email accounts passwords, revenue accounts like Amazon and eBay, etc., blogs access are a few examples) information.

It's important to understand that this <u>does not mean they have or need access</u> to our money or our stuff. Generally this person is going to be the power of attorney for our healthcare and finances (there are legal documents to create and designate these) anyway, and we are the ones who determine when control of our stuff gets turned over to them.

Therefore, it's important to pick someone we trust and it's important to review those documents from time to time to ensure that all the information is updated. People get divorced. People die. We add and we drop banks, policies, jobs all the times. Make sure your legal documents reflect all of these.

On insurance policies, be sure to name an actual person as a beneficiary instead of having your estate as the beneficiary. If the estate is the beneficiary, then everything has to go to probate, which can be a lengthy legal process, before the funds needed to pay whatever outstanding debts you have are available. No one wants to leave those behind with that kind of financial mess.

At this step, then, in the progression of dementias and Alzheimer's disease, our main concern is the health and welfare of our loved ones. Since we know their wishes and we, often, are the ones who are responsible for making sure those wishes are adhered to, then our loved ones wishes must guide everything related to their medical care.

Let's talk about some of the areas of medical care that come into play here:

1. Keeping our loved ones involved in the discussions and decisions related to medical care

    Whether our loved ones with dementias and Alzheimer's Disease are fully able to participate in and understand everything about their medical care, it is important that we include them in every aspect and do our best to communicate what is going on to them. The worst thing that we can do is talk and make decisions about medical care as if they're not even in the room.

    They may not fully understand, but this is a matter of honor and dignity in recognizing that as long as they are alive, they are not invisible and we're not taking over their lives (even though we often have to make the final decisions, but they must be made within the scope of what our loved ones have communicated to us that they want or don't want).

2. Establishing the limits of medical care

    A point comes when medical care will do more harm than good or present risks that outweigh positive outcomes. One of these is surgical procedures.

    There are many risks related to surgeries for our loved ones with dementias and Alzheimer's Disease. Even if our loved ones are physically healthy, surgical procedures can accelerate and deepen the neurological decline, especially with the use of general anesthesia. Most dementias and Alzheimer's Disease patients who undergo surgery under general anesthesia experience a significant and permanent decline in cognitive function from where they were before the surgery.

If our loved ones have physical health problems in addition to dementias and Alzheimer's Disease, then whether to do surgical procedures and under what circumstances must be weighed in light of that.

For example, my mom's medical profile included vascular dementia, Lewy body dementia, Alzheimer's Disease, chronic and hard-to-control hypertension, and congestive heart failure.

Five and a half months before her death, she was in a lot of pain – it was in her lower right torso – and was vomiting, sweating but cold and clammy to the touch, and pale.

Unsure of whether it was her heart, I told Mom I thought we should go to the hospital and get her checked out. Mom agreed after a few hours of these symptoms. She had an infected gall bladder.

Mom was admitted and we both awoke early the next morning to a gastrointestinal surgeon who wanted to put her under general anesthesia and remove the gall bladder.

I said, "No." Mom's congestive heart failure, by then, was worsening by the day, and I knew that her heart couldn't take the procedure. I asked him about alternatives to remove the infection without general anesthesia.

The surgeon literally rolled his eyes and sucked his teeth before telling me that the only alternative was to administer antibiotics and use a local anesthetic to insert a drain for six weeks to pull the infection out, "But," he said, "If the gall bladder isn't removed, this infection could come back in a year or two."

I knew by then that Mom didn't have a year or two left, so I talked with Mom and explained the drain and antibiotics and she agreed to that, so I told the surgeon that's what we would do.

He wasn't happy with the decision – and I had to get him to change the paperwork the next morning before I would sign it because he'd done paperwork for removing the gall bladder under general anesthesia – but I made the decision based on what was best for Mom.

After that hospitalization, which was hard on Mom and me, Mom said she didn't want to go back to the hospital ever again. And we honored her wishes, which was how hospice got involved when she began having the more frequent chest pains that culminated in a major heart attack.

3. Advocating for our loved ones

   Our loved ones with dementias and Alzheimer's Disease
   are no longer in a position to fully and adequately
   advocate for themselves with regard to medical care.

   In general, the medical profession tends to run
   roughshod (much of this has to do with making a profit
   and being in bed with pharmaceutical companies and
   insurance companies) over all the people who pay their
   salaries. It's just the nature of the beast it has become.

   However, because of their neurological impairments, our
   loved ones are even more vulnerable to this and they are
   in no position to do anything about it.

   That's where we come in. While our loved ones continue
   to dictate the amount and level of their care, we're the
   ones who communicate that and approve or disapprove
   what medical professionals are proposing.

   In addition, to properly treat our loved ones with
   dementias and Alzheimer's Disease, an accurate health
   summary must be provided with each medical visit. This
   includes up-to-date medication lists (the primary care
   physician can and should provide an updated list with
   each office visit), vital signs, and a complete description
   of recurring, worsening, or new medical issues since the
   last visit.

It is our responsibility to know this, stay on top this, and provide this on each visit to a medical facility.

This is especially critical in admissions to the hospital, where the trend is increasingly moving toward hospitalists who strictly work for the hospital – and, therefore, have no knowledge of and no relationship with their patients - instead of primary care physicians having access to their patients and control over their care during hospital stays.

And this is very useful when our loved ones have home health or palliative care services, because it helps the nurses to adequately and accurately guide care needs and changes.

4. Handling hospitalizations

Being in the hospital is hard on anyone, but it is especially hard on our loved ones with dementias and Alzheimer's Disease for several reasons.

The first is simply that they are in a strange place, their routines are turned upside down, and they are continually encountering and interacting with new and strange people. It is very common for our loved ones to be more confused, more agitated, and more disagreeable in general during hospital stays.

Another reason why hospitalizations are hard on our loved ones with dementias and Alzheimer's Disease is because they don't get individualized and personal 24/7 care. Nurses pop in once in a while, doctors show up whenever, and CNA staffing is often either low or the ratio of patients is too high. Therefore, the basic needs of our loves are not met often enough or, at times, not at all.

We should be at the hospital when our loved ones are in the hospital. This means spending the night in those uncomfortable chairs with a thin blanket and lumpy pillow – if we're lucky – and being there during the day to advocate for health care decisions, to discuss treatment options with our loved ones, and to help meet their basic needs when there are no hospital staff available.

It's a major pain. I will admit that, having had to do just that quite a bit over the last twelve years of my mom's life.

But it's a small price to pay to be there to give the help to our loved ones with dementias and Alzheimer's that they need, to be actively involved with, advocating for, and communicating with them about their care, and, most importantly, to be that familiar face that gives them a measure of comfort, stability, familiarity, and love in a totally unfamiliar environment.

It's a gift. We should be willing to give it. No matter how much we have to. No matter how often.

5. Getting home health care and palliative care

    After each hospitalization that our loved ones with Alzheimer's Disease and dementias has, we should secure home health care to follow up at home before they are released.

    Home health care is provided to patients who have an acute skill need – such as heart disease, a stroke, or uncontrolled high blood pressure – in the comfort and privacy of their homes without the need for endless doctor's visits. Medicare covers home health services for the duration of the need.

    In addition to providing nursing visits on a weekly basis, home health agencies also provide occupational therapy, physical therapy, and speech therapy. All of these can be quite beneficial to our loved ones with dementias and Alzheimer's Disease and we should take advantage of the ones that fit the needs that our loved ones have.

    Once the acute skill need no longer exists, then most home health agencies offer palliative care services. This doesn't require an acute skill, but is basically a maintenance program of home health services, including nursing and all the therapies listed above, for as long as our loved ones need them.

Primary care physicians write the orders for palliative care services and the request can generally be made over the phone or through the nurse at the home health care agency.

The same professionals that offer home health services offer palliative care services, so there is a continuity of service for our loved ones with dementias and Alzheimer's Disease.

I highly recommend asking that the same staff do all the visits. This is the least disruptive way to provide these services to our loved ones because the same people come to our homes all the time and a trust and comfort level between them and our loved ones develops.

The great benefit to having home health care and palliative care is more evident as our loved ones with dementias and Alzheimer's Disease progress in their neurological impairment because having these services basically eliminates in-office doctor's visits. Additionally, the nursing staff is often able to get action taken quickly on physical needs that need urgent attention when we as personal advocates for our loved ones may have a very hard time getting things added, eliminated or changed.

A word of advice on choosing your home health care provider. Often times, hospitals partner with a specific home health agency and that will be the agency that initially provides services to our loved ones with dementias and Alzheimer's Disease.

However, if we and/or our loved ones are unhappy with the agency, then we can fire them and bring our own agency in (this will require the primary care physician writing orders for the new agency).

We should never settle for bad service or inferior service. We should never settle for disregard, disrespect, or disinterest toward our loved ones with dementias and Alzheimer's Disease.

Research the home health agencies in your area. Visit or talk to them on the phone (generally the first phone call is enough to let you know whether you want to use them or not – a lot of these agencies have some incredibly rude and dismissive people on their staff and they are likely to end up as your first point of contact).

It's also important to be aware that all home health agencies offer, at a minimum, home health care and hospice services. These are two separate departments within the agencies (they can seem like two separate agencies sometimes), staffed by entirely different people.

Although we'll talk about hospice in depth in a later chapter, you need to know that you don't have to use the hospice services of the agency that provides you with home health services.

It's a good idea to start talking to different hospice services as well and determine which one will be the one to provide end-of-life care for your loved ones when they are at the point where they will need hospice services.

Remember, if you don't like them when you make initial contact with them, then you're going to like them even less when your loved ones and you are going through the dying process and need a lot of help and support.

As our loved ones with dementias and Alzheimer's Disease progress through their journeys, they reach this step where their dignity and their independence could be compromised. It is our job to ensure that we preserve their dignity to the end and ensure as much independence as is safe to the end.

Dignity is something that all human beings should have until they take their last breath. This includes respect and honor toward them, no matter what circumstances they may find themselves in. It is no different for our loved ones with dementias and Alzheimer's Disease.

In addition to dignity, it is also important for us to ensure that our loved ones have as much independence – guaranteeing safety at all times – over their own bodies and their own care as they are able to handle.

It will take them longer and everything may not be perfect, but as long as our loved ones with dementias and Alzheimer's Disease can participate in their care, their lives, and our lives safely, the more happy and satisfied they will be and the more dignity and honor we will be showing them.

What does this look like in practice?

1. Incontinence and toileting

   When our loved ones reach this step, we may begin to have to help them with toileting. Generally, urinary incontinence is the first toileting issue we encounter. This may be due more to age and medication than the actual loss of urinary continence, so our loved ones will likely know they need to urinate, but just not be able to make it in time.

We want the transition to adult incontinence clothing to be as easy and stigma-free for them as possible, so we should treat the clothing, accidents, and any other issues we encounter with no fuss and calmly and normally.

For example, my mom had continence issues the last few years of her life because of the diuretics she was taking for congestive heart failure. She knew, right up until the end of her life, when she needed to go to the bathroom. But because of her own slowing down and the decreased ability to hold it, she often didn't make it to the bathroom in time when the diuretics kicked in.

She began wearing protective undergarments – I always called them "panties" – when she became aware of the problem, especially when we were traveling or would be out of the house for a while. Eventually, she wore them all the time.

There were times when Mom would have accidents and would really get upset about it and those were the times when I reassured her that it was no big deal and that we had electricity, a washer and a dryer, and detergent, so cleaning up and taking care of it wasn't a problem. That always kept her distress to a minimum and it also maintained her dignity and her respect, even in a situation that was personally embarrassing to her.

As time went on, I began to have to help Mom with other toileting activities, but because I did it with no muss and no fuss, it preserved Mom's dignity in spite of the fact that someone else was involved in helping her do things she'd always been able to do by herself.

2. Bathing and personal grooming

One of the ways that we can ensure that our loved ones with dementia and Alzheimer's Disease maintain both their dignity and independence is in the areas of bathing and personal grooming.

We should always be attentive to encouraging and letting our loved ones do as much as they are able for themselves in these two areas, no matter how much of an active role we have to take in ensuring cleanliness and neatness.

If our loved ones are able to bathe themselves, then we should by all means let them do anything they are able to. However, it may be that we have to help when safety – the possibility of falling or limited mobility – becomes an issue. But anything they are able to continue to do, we should encourage them to do.

My mom could handle most of her bathing until the last eight months of her life. As she grew weaker and falling became a greater risk, I began to help Mom more, but continued to encourage her to do as much as she was able on her own. Near the end of Mom's life, the only bathing she could do without my help was washing her face, so I made sure to hand her the soapy washcloth twice a day so that she could wash her face.

Mom could do most of her personal grooming until the end of her life, so after I'd put the toothpaste on her toothbrush, I'd stand behind her, holding on to her while she brushed her teeth twice a day. I'd do the same while she was brushing her hair after I washed it.

I had begun cutting Mom's fingernails and toenails early after her diagnoses, simply because it became harder for her to figure out how to use the clippers. One of the things that I introduced was something I have never personally done for myself, but that gave Mom an opportunity to do something for herself with regard to the care of her fingernails.

I taught Mom how to put clear nail polish on her own nails – I removed it every couple weeks and then we'd repeat the process. This gave Mom an active role in her personal grooming and it made this activity enjoyable and it gave us some bonding time, which was priceless.

I will mention here that taking care of our loved ones' skin is an important part of personal grooming. As skin ages, it gets thinner and it becomes rougher. A lot of the commercial body washes and soaps on the market actually dry out the skin, especially if used every day.

So, in an effort to keep our loved ones skin as healthy as possible, a good recommendation is to bathe with soap and water every other day and use pre-moistened (preferably with aloe) adult washcloths to clean up the other days. Liberally apply a good-quality lotion every day and use facial moisturizers every day. Not only is this calming and soothing, but it keeps skin soft and pliable and comfortable for our loved ones.

Two other things that are important with bathing are privacy and temperature. Always bathe in a private area, whether that's in the bathroom or a separate room. Our loved ones deserve that privacy.

Be sure that wherever bathing is taking place that the temperature is warm and comfortable. Because my only full bathroom was upstairs and Mom couldn't get upstairs, her bathing happened in the kitchen.

About half an hour before Mom's bath, I'd take a chair, all her clothes, and a towel and a wash cloth into the kitchen, along with soap and shampoo. I had a large heater just for the kitchen and I'd turn it on high to get the kitchen, which was large and airy and, therefore, cooler than the rest of the house, toasty and warm so Mom would be comfortable during her bath.

On the days we did the pre-moistened adult washcloth baths, we did those in the bathroom and I would make sure the bathroom was warm and toasty as well.

These are little touches, but they are signs of our respect and honor and care for and about our loved ones. The littlest things, in our minds, are probably the greatest ways we show them love. Never forget that.

3. Dressing

As with toileting, bathing, and personal grooming, we should encourage and let our loved ones with dementias and Alzheimer's Disease participate in dressing themselves as much as they are able and as is safe.

It's almost second-nature to start taking over and doing everything for our loved ones because it's faster if we do it ourselves. However, we shouldn't do this for two reasons.

One is that our loved ones with dementias and Alzheimer's Disease will pick up on our "hurrying" and it may trigger confusion, anxiety, and agitation. It may also trigger the feeling that they're an inconvenience or are standing in the way of something we should be doing or want to do. That is the last thing that we want to convey to our loved ones. So we should always be willing to slow down to their pace and take whatever time they need to get dressed.

The second reason is that the more we do for our loved ones that they can do for themselves, the more independence they lose. At some point, the "fight" to do what they can for themselves becomes too tiring and too much effort for our loved ones if we constantly take over and brush their attempts aside, and they will give up even trying to do anything.

We never ever want to do that to our loved ones with dementias and Alzheimer's Disease. Yes, these diseases are fatal. Yes, these diseases steal independence slowly from our loved ones. Yes, the day may come, if our loved ones live long enough, when they actually will not be able to do anything for themselves. But we don't want to take that ability and that independence from them as long as they have it because of our impatience and thoughtlessness.

4. Helping with daily activities

We have discussed this in other chapters, but in this one, we'll focus on the dignity and independence aspects of encouraging and letting our loved ones with dementias and Alzheimer's Disease help as much as they are able and as is safe with the daily activities of living.

By including our loved ones in the daily activities of life, we are showing them that they are needed, that their contributions are important, and that they are a vital part of our lives and our families.

Just as our parents began to include us when we were young in family activities such as gardening, household chores, and taking care of pets, we need to encourage and include our loved ones with dementias and Alzheimer's Disease in these same activities now.

It may be just sitting in the kitchen with us at the table while we do prep work for a meal. It may be helping us water plants. It may be helping us fold laundry. It may be any of a number of manageable things for them to participate in, but by including them and giving them something to do, we give them meaning and purpose in their lives and we maintain their dignity and their independence as much as we're able.

Chapter 13: "And Know They Love You"

At this step, and indeed throughout the entire journey of dementias and Alzheimer's Disease, we must always make sure that our loved ones know the we love them, we care about them, and we are committed to them.

As our loved ones become more dependent on us and as they lose cognition and neurological function, they often become fearful. Their fears include being isolated, being abandoned, being a burden, and being in the way. For those who are still able to communicate at this step, much of their conversations with us will include these fears.

It is our job to allay those fears and remind our loved ones with dementias and Alzheimer's Disease that we're on their side and we're not going anywhere. Spending a lot of time with them becomes more critical at this step as do what we do with our loved ones during that time together.

How can we demonstrate our love, our commitment, our care and our concern in tangible ways?

1. Quality time

   One of the most reassuring things that we can do for our loved ones with dementias and Alzheimer's Disease is to spend quality time with them. This is not just spending time, but it is time where our attention is completely dedicated to them.

   While quality time can include some sort of fun or interesting activities, more often than not, it is just being with them and listening to them, interacting with them, and giving them our undivided attention.

2. Conversations

As I mentioned, many of the conversations that we have with our loved ones with dementias and Alzheimer's Disease at this step will include things they are afraid of or worried about. Much of this will be centered on their concerns and how they think or believe they are negatively impacting our lives.

One of the things my mom said to me quite often as she neared the end of her life was that she didn't want to be a burden on me. More than once she told me I ought to just put her "away some place," and get back to living my life.

I knew that somewhere inside Mom knew that my decision to take care of her was going to have consequences for me after she was gone. I knew it was going to have consequences for me after she was gone (I had no idea it would turn out to be what it has turned out to be, but I would do it all over again exactly the way I did it, because it was the right thing to do and I loved Mom enough to put my life on the line).

And here's what I also knew. Mom had given up a career to adopt children and raise them, with my dad, as her own. That decision was hard on her and my dad physically, emotionally, and mentally, but there was never a doubt that they were committed, they loved us, and they'd do it all over again in spite of what it cost them.

And this was my opportunity to thank Mom and to give back to her what she and my dad had given me. Not in full, because there's no way a child can ever do a full return on the investment his or her parents have made in him or her. I saw it, at best, as a down payment on all I had received from them.

It also gave Mom and me the opportunity to spend the last years of her life together. I could never stomach the idea of entrusting Mom's care to people who didn't know her, didn't love her, and who didn't care about her the way I did it. Even though I made more than my fair share of mistakes taking care of Mom, I loved her and that love was the driving force behind everything I did.

So when we had these conversations, I would recall for Mom all that she and my dad had done for us kids. I would tell the stories back to her that she used to tell us of our early days on the planet. I'd tell family stories from our entire history together.

And then I would tell her that I loved her and she wasn't a burden. I'd tell her that I wasn't going to put her away some place. I'd tell her that I was going to be with her every step of the way and she wouldn't be alone. And I'd reassure her that everything would be okay with me after she was gone.

We had a lot of these conversations, and each time, as I listened, as I responded, as I reassured Mom, I could see the palpable relief that she'd been heard, that she was safe, and that she was loved.

That, my friends, was priceless. To and for both of us.

3. Embraces, holding hands, and kisses

There is no stronger way to say "I love you" to our loved ones with dementias and Alzheimer's Disease than what we can express through touch. All human beings – even introverts like me, although I'm a little weird sometimes about who I want in my space, touching me, and for how long – need touch.

In the late 19th century, a German foundling home, in which physical touch between the staff and children was absolutely forbidden, had a mortality rate of more than 70% of its infants under the age of one. American orphanages in the early 20th century, which had the same prohibition on touch, had mortality rates that averaged 53% in children under two years of age.

The absence or presence of touch, in the intervening years, has been scientifically researched and proven to cause a failure to thrive or to induce thriving.

That need for touch is no less imperative for our loved ones suffering from dementias and Alzheimer's Disease.

I've been in a lot of nursing homes over the course of my life, mainly as a volunteer, and I am convinced that both a lack of physical touch, as well as the sometimes rough and exasperated painful touching of staff who clearly see their responsibilities as a bother or an inconvenience (there are some good folks in these places, but they tend not to stay long because of what they see and experience as staff, and the ones who aren't good tend to be entrenched), are reasons why elderly folks often shrivel up quickly and die once they are moved to one of these facilities.

So what can we do for our loved ones with dementias and Alzheimer's Disease? Maintaining physical contact throughout the day is a key part of showing our love, our care, and our concern to them. It should be gentle, kind, comforting and reassuring.

One of the ways we can do this is through embraces. We can put our arms around them and hold them close and we can hug them. Holding our loved ones and letting them hold us is soothing all the way around. I don't care how old a child gets, there's nothing like being hugged and held by your parents. There is no substitute. The same goes true for our parents getting hugged and held by us.

Another way that we can give our loved ones with dementias and Alzheimer's Disease the gift of touch is through holding their hands.

And a third way we can give this gift of touch to our loved ones is through kisses on the cheek.

Mom and I did all of these often through the day and sometimes through the night if both of us were up, but we had a morning and nightly routine that never wavered.

Each night when I tucked Mom into bed, I'd hug her, kiss her on both cheeks, and I'd say, "I love you; good night and sleep tight." Then I'd take her hearing aids out and put them away and pat her on the shoulder as she started to drift on to sleep.

Each morning, I was up before Mom was. I would say my prayers, then grab some coffee and would sit in the dark room with her and watch the news until she woke up. As soon as Mom woke up, I'd go over and hug her and kiss her and I'd say, "Good morning!"

Those were two special times for both of us each day and I believe it made a world of difference in how well Mom did in spite of her dementias, Alzheimer's Disease, and congestive heart failure right up to the day she died.

Chapter 14: "As the Final Curtain Falls Before My Eyes"

This step is the next to the last step in the journey that our loved ones with dementias and Alzheimer's Disease take. It can be a lengthy step of months or a short step of weeks or a shorter step of just few days. Regardless of the amount of time, though, this step is harder, I believe, on us than it is on our loved ones.

This step is a two-process step: the body begins shutting down in the first process and active dying occurs in the second process.

One of the first signs that the body is beginning to shut down that we'll see with our loved ones with dementias and Alzheimer's Disease is that they will start sleeping a lot more.

This usually begins a few months before death occurs. Often, this is a pattern of an hour or two of wakefulness followed by naps and dozing on and off during the day, with fatigue setting in early in the evening and a full night's sleep ensuing.

In short, our loved ones will be asleep more than they are awake.

Another sign may be a decreased desire for food and drink. It is important to not to try to force food and liquids on our loved ones with dementias and Alzheimer's Disease if they don't want them. As the body starts its elaborate shutdown process, there simply isn't a need for much nourishment. Additionally, because our loved ones are not very active, they don't burn a lot of calories nor do they need as much sustenance.

However, what is also likely to happen is that our loved ones will want or need nourishment at odd times of the day (not necessarily a normal meal time), and when they do, try to keep food and drinks healthy and light (easy to digest).

Often, during this time of shutting down, our loved ones with dementias and Alzheimer's Disease will, when they are awake, both sort through their lives and work to make peace with anything in their pasts that they believe is left unsettled.

There were two things that stood out in conversations my mom and I had when she was going through this step.

One was that, even at the end of her life, Mom was still trying to answer basic questions about the early years of her life. Mom lost both parents by the age of six and lived for the twelve years after that with an aunt who, along with her immediate family, was unloving and unaffectionate and made it clear that Mom wasn't wanted there. This aunt, at times, could also be very abusive, very hateful, and very cruel.

Many of Mom's conversations during this time ended up on this subject and the core question she'd never found the answer to was the one Mom asked each time: "Why did they hate me so much?" We'd always talk about it and I would remind Mom that the time was coming when all that would be fixed and that although we might not have the answers now, one day the answers would come.

The second thing that Mom talked about a lot was all the people she'd loved who had died. I learned more about how deeply those deaths had affected her and how great the losses had been for her.

One conversation in particular struck me the last full week Mom was alive when she started talking about someone named Jimmy and how much she loved him and how deeply it broke her heart when he died.

During the conversation, I just listened because, at the time, I didn't know who Mom was talking about, but this was a brand new revelation about Mom's pain that I didn't know about until then.

It wasn't until early the next morning when I was lying awake in the dark that I realized that Jimmy was one of Mom's younger cousins who had died in a tractor accident just before his 17th birthday.

I'd always know that Mom had been close to Jimmy and his brother, but she had never revealed how profoundly his life and his death affected her. Mom had just never talked about it before.

The best thing that we can do is to listen and provide comfort and reassurance during their conversations. We need to our loved ones with dementias and Alzheimer's Disease talk, even if it's repetitive, painful, or hard to listen to. This is part of the process of dying.

Toward the end of the shutdown process, our loved ones may express a desire to see family and/or friends (dead and living). This is part of the letting-go process, so we need to make sure that family and/or friends know that time is getting short and if they want to be there, they need to be there sooner rather than later.

Be aware that everyone handles the dying process differently. Some people will come and some people won't come. That's life, but getting all caught in that and getting upset about it if they choose not to come only hurts our loved ones who need us to be present, supportive, and comforting.

Each person has to live with the decision he or she makes as to how they deal with our loved ones' end of life process and we are not in anyone else's shoes but our own, so it's imperative that we stay focused on our loved ones with dementias and Alzheimer's Disease and not condemn or ascribe motives to others about the decisions they make.

Palliative care will continue through this shutdown process, but a point will come when the transition to hospice care will need to occur.

Let's talk about hospice now. To be admitted to hospice, our loved ones have to meet all the diagnostic criteria for that admission. The diagnostic criteria for admission to hospice under dementias and Alzheimer's Disease is, in my opinion, ridiculous because our loved ones can't be admitted under that diagnosis until they are already in the process of actively dying.

Also, once admitted to hospice under a diagnosis, there can be no more medical treatment for that medical issue (no hospitals, no doctors, no medical intervention at all), so it's important to not admit our loved ones too soon or under a diagnosis that needs to be medically treated for the time being.

With Mom, in addition to the dementias and Alzheimer's Disease, congestive heart failure was also a medical condition we were dealing with acutely on a chronic basis.

Mom complained almost every day for the last three months of her life of pain across her shoulders and sometimes in her chest. We were increasing the diuretics at least once a week because Mom was retaining too much fluid. I knew her aortic valve replacement was eight years past the 10-year warranty the cardiac surgeon had given Dad, Mom, and me when we had the consultation to decide which valve Mom would get.

So I knew Mom's heart was the time bomb that was ticking the fastest. Because we'd had the no-more-hospitals conversation – which, for my own peace of mind, I would ask and confirm with Mom each time she told me about these pains that she didn't want to go to the hospital – I knew that would probably be the leading culprit in her death. Mom would agree and I knew we were on the same page.

One morning in early August, Mom woke up with chest pains. I called home health and they told me to take her to the hospital. I said we weren't doing hospitals anymore. They said they would send a nurse out.

They sent a nurse and the hospice director. The hospice director told Mom and me it was time to admit her to hospice for heart disease. Neither Mom nor I had an opportunity to really discuss it or think about it because I knew the gravity of the situation with Mom's heart, so we both agreed to it.

Had I had more time to prepare, I would have chosen a different hospice agency. Mom and I had met with this hospice director several months before because we wanted to talk about their hospice program and when would be the right time to consider hospice.

Making the decision for hospice is an emotional decision in a lot of ways because it is a recognition that life is coming to an end. I am a pragmatic person and not overly emotional about doing what needs to be done or has to be done, but I expected a measure of empathy and consolation in that decision-making process.

The hospice director, in that first meeting, was distant, lacked empathy, and was anything but consoling. I decided then that I wouldn't go with that hospice agency and talked to some nurses I knew and got the name of another agency that was considered the best in the area.

But on that Wednesday morning, when Mom was having chest pains, and I knew something had to be done then, when that same hospice director was in our living room, I agreed to go with the home health agency's hospice group.

It was the right decision because the next evening, after we'd received our hospice package earlier that day, Mom had a major heart attack, and, by having hospice in place, I was able to administer the medications she needed and direct the firemen that came to help me get Mom to bed not to do anything more than move her.

It may be that, as was the case with my mom, the home health staff is, for the most part, great, but the hospice staff is not great or just awful. If you have a hospice agency that you don't like or is not doing a good job (ours didn't for that first week, but fortunately, the saving grace was, after a week, that a home health nurse filling in for a hospice nurse agreed to be our nurse with Mom through the end), then you have the right to fire them and get another agency.

If our loved ones are at a point where changing will mean no care for them when they need it most, then we have the right to ask for different staff. Don't be shy and don't hesitate if hospice is not meeting our loved ones' needs. This is about our loved ones with dementias and Alzheimer's Disease and their end of life, not about whether the hospice agency is going to get upset or somebody's going to get their feelings hurt. We have to do what's best for our loved ones.

Mom recovered somewhat from the heart attack, but she was much weaker and I knew a lot of damage had been done and the heart attack had had taken its toll on her. Mom slept for almost 48 hours straight after the heart attack, and I wasn't sure we weren't at the end of life for her then. But after sleeping that long, Mom woke up and was alert and, although much slower, she was able to walk a little and go through our normal daily activities to some degree.

But, I knew something was different and I knew in the back of my mind that Mom's life was winding down toward the end.

Mom began the active dying process on the day that she rallied spectacularly – rallies like this are not uncommon and are an incredible gift if we get them – when, after a week of not knowing who I was, she recognized me. My sister had come in from out of town and we had an incredible day of conversations, laughter, memories, and love.

But Mom, who was still taking diuretics and was eating and drinking pretty normally, was urinating very little that day. I told my sister that I thought her kidneys were shutting down and if Mom was dry when she got up the next morning that I was going to call the hospice nurse to check her out.

Mom woke up the next morning alert, happy, and bone dry. I called the hospice nurse. The nurse came and said Mom looked good and to keep an eye on her urine output during the day and she'd come back by the house that night.

We ate breakfast after the nurse left and then Mom told us she was tired and wanted to take a little nap. We both kissed her and tucked her into her chair and she dozed off.

Mom woke up a few hours later and she was, I realized later, afraid. I don't even know that Mom recognized my sister or me. We got her some yogurt and something to drink and sat down with her. Mom ate the yogurt, but knocked the cup of water away when I tried to give it to her and shook her head.

Mom said she was hurting and when I asked where, she moved her hand across her chest. I got the smaller dose of morphine and gave it to Mom and waited a few minutes before asking her if it helped. Mom said it was still hurting. I gave her another small dose of morphine and she looked at my sister and me and that's when she said, "I guess they're going to throw me out now."

I took Mom's hands and held them and told her that she was home, nobody was going to throw her out, and we were right there with her.

My sister opened a photo album and Mom started turning the pages with one hand while I held her other hand. The only person she recognized was my dad in the first few pages, but then she closed her eyes and went to sleep still turning the blank pages.

Mom never woke up again, even though she was still alive. The hospice nurse stopped back by that night, as promised, and she was shocked at the change in Mom.

Mom had fallen asleep in a chair and the three of us moved her into bed. The nurse put a catheter in and told us that Mom was dying and we needed to keep her comfortable.

She gave us a morphine schedule and told us to stop all other medication. She also said not to worry about vital signs - I had gotten so used to taking those several times a

day that that particular thing was hard for me to let go of –
and to make sure to keep Mom's mouth moist.

She said our home health nurse would be back the next day,
if we didn't call or need them before then.

A little over 48 hours later, Mom took her last breath. It was
a very peaceful death. Mom was comfortable with the
morphine, and we kept her cleaned up, her mouth moist,
and we made sure she wasn't uncomfortable temperature-
wise, even though it was August and hotter-than-usual
August at that.

Our hospice nurse had visited a couple of hours before Mom
died and he told us that death was a matter of hours away.
We'd spent the day with Mom, singing hymns, talking to her,
and me reading the Bible to her, reminding her that it was
almost over and we'd see Dad and her again soon. We
reminded her that we loved her.

My sister and I had left the room for no more than 30
seconds when Mom died. We walked back in together and as
I saw Mom's face, I asked the question I already knew the
answer to: "Is Mom dead?"

Chapter 15: "I Have a Lock of Hair and One-Half of My Heart"

Death and its aftermath is the last step of this journey through dementias and Alzheimer's Disease and it is a step that we take without our loved ones.

It is often said that in these neurological and fatal diseases that we experience death twice. The first death is the loss of the loved ones we knew before these diseases. The second death is when our loved ones take their last breath.

If hospice is on board, the first phone call we make is to them. A nurse will come out and confirm death. Hospice will also contact the funeral home and will prepare the body for transport. This includes cleaning and dressing (I actually helped our hospice nurse with this).

When the people from the funeral home get there, they will make an appointment to come in and make burial arrangements (usually the next day) and they will take the body to the funeral home and start the embalming process.

Once the funeral home people leave, the hospice nurse will collect and destroy any remaining medications and there will be paperwork to sign both to confirm the medication disposal and to end hospice services.

It's a flurry of activity that lasts several hours, and I personally found that to be just what I needed because the reality that Mom was gone was still sinking in.

The next phase is the funeral and the burial arrangements, and then the funeral and burial itself. Although Mom's death sunk in quickly, because I was directing and coordinating everything leading up to the funeral and burial, I didn't have time to linger on or sort through what Mom's death really meant to me and for me.

It wasn't until everyone that had come into town for the services left and just my sister and I were there alone that I finally had any kind of opportunity to confront what life looked like without Mom.

But, even then, there were thank you notes, returning things to the medical equipment company, getting Mom's clothes together and donating them to a local abused women's shelter, making sure that the gravestone folks would get out to the graveyard and updated the double gravestone that marked where Dad and Mom were buried with Mom's date of death, getting all the family photo albums sent to a scanner to be scanned and put on DVD for everyone, paying any outstanding bills, and, of course, notifying the agencies I needed to about Mom's death.

Once my sister left, though, was when the full impact of Mom's death hit me. The house was deafeningly quiet. When Mom was alive, I was going pretty much 24/7, but now that she was gone, I suddenly had almost nothing to do.

Each time I walked by the chair where Mom spent a lot of time - it had been my dad's chair before that - I would touch it and an emerging hole in my heart would get a little bigger.

I'd always kept the bathroom light on at night so that Mom wouldn't be afraid if and when she woke up during the night and so that she could see that I was right there beside her. It took a month before I could bring myself to turn that light off at night, even though I was sleeping back in my bed upstairs.

Grief edged in slowly, but deeply. I found myself taking an inventory of my entire life and rehashing, analyzing, going over in minute detail everything I'd done – or hadn't done – right.

It descended into something I'm still not completely out of yet: a thorough thrashing of myself for all the things I hadn't known, I didn't do, I should have done, or I shouldn't have done.

I realized what Mom had gone through after Dad died only after Mom died. I regretted not moving back here after his death so Mom wouldn't have been all alone.

Now that I was all alone, I understood how hard it must have been for her. I couldn't believe that I didn't know what I didn't know and I had a lot of guilt about not knowing it.

Practically speaking, I couldn't have known it or really understood it then, but I was still angry with myself for not knowing or understanding it.

Grief expanded until it overwhelmed me. I was working, going through the motions, but inside I was in pain, much like I remembered going through when my dad died, but somehow even more intense because, I think, my last parent was gone and I didn't have anybody in that role left to turn to.

I have never felt more alone in the world than I have in the time since Mom died. I never can – and won't be able to here either – explain that in tangible terms that make sense to anybody else.

I have acquaintances. I have friends. I have family. And yet I, in the physical sense, feel totally alone.

Perhaps it was because Mom and I, in spite of the differences in our personalities and temperaments, were always close and she and Daddy were the two people I could count on being there for me no matter what.

They and she didn't always understand me, but they never didn't not love me. You know, there's that unwritten rule some place that parents have to love you no matter what. And mine did.

And for that first time in my life, that unconditional, guaranteed human love that I could count on, that I depended on, that I needed was gone. And I didn't know what to do without that.

It seemed as time went on and the further out from Mom's death I got, the stronger the grief, the stronger the emotions, and the stronger the pain. I know it should have been the opposite, but that's not the way it worked with me.

The world also seemed to get darker and emptier and I became more and more of a stranger in the midst of a rhythm of life that didn't make any sense to me.

I couldn't understand how people could be happy, be unconcerned, and be so frivolous. I felt more and more isolated from the human race.

I turned to God in tears more than I didn't and asked for forgiveness and healing and help. Although it was often on my knees, it was just as often at any given moment when everything came crashing in on me and tears turned into sobbing and sobbing turned into pleas for forgiveness.

Everything emotionally in me has seemed to rise to live just underneath my skin and it takes just a word or a phrase or some innocuous comment for it to pop to the surface and reduce me to tears.

What has been maddening for me is that I've always been an emotional stuffer.

I always have seen being emotional as being weak and out of control (actually, with all this I have and do see myself as weak and out of control, fortunately just privately, but it's very uncomfortable for me to deal with and live with).

So, for me, the best way to handle emotions is not to. Stuff it inside and go on.

You probably already know where I'm going before you get there.

Apparently, there's a limit to how much emotion you can stuff inside before it starts making its way back up and out.

And there's nothing like the trigger of death to make the outflowing trickle turn into a lava-spewing, ash-covering, life-altering volcano that makes Italy's Mt. Vesuvius (considered one of the world's deadliest volcanos, after an eruption in 79 A.D. almost instantly killed over 16,000 people in Pompeii) volcano seem like a tiny backyard fire pit.

But in and through all this I have some lessons to pass on to you.

Grief is a process and it takes time to get through the process. All days won't be horrible days, but all days won't be good days either.

The grief process seems to run in cycles that alternate between intense pain and intense numbness. Either you feel everything or you feel absolutely nothing. There doesn't seem to be any in between.

Give yourself that time. You can't quit living in the process, but be prepared for it to not feel good or feel normal for a very long time. If it was any way other than that, then there would be no love, no care, no concern, no connection between and for us as people.

Don't let yourself get stuck in a "would've, should've, could've" mindset. None of us go through this journey with our loved ones with dementias and Alzheimer's Disease without making mistakes, without times when we don't understand, without moments that we wished hadn't happened or that we could have prevented.

There will be a period of time somewhere in the grieving process where this mindset is the only one you've got and it has the capability, if it doesn't have a finite beginning and a finite end, to drive you insane. Don't let it.

At some point, you have to let go and move on. The longer you linger here, the more unhealthy it will be for you. I'm not saying not to stop for it, because it's part of the process. What I am saying is not to let it be the last stop in the process.

Don't be angry or upset with people who haven't been through this journey and don't understand what it was or what its aftermath is.

Just as we don't know what we don't know as we go through the steps of this journey of dementias and Alzheimer's Disease with our loved ones, people who have never been through it don't know what they don't know.

Be kind and patient with them, even if they're not always kind and patient with you. Be forgiving of ignorance, of lack of knowledge, of not understanding. I'm not saying it's easy. It is not! But this is an imperative for us.

Pray and ask for healing and peace. This journey is not always a peaceful one when we're going through it with our loved ones, and the process of grieving can open up a lot of old wounds – and some new ones – and can be, at times, anything but peaceful. That's why we need to ask God for healing and for peace, because it's not going to come any other way.

And last, don't waste the pain. For those of us who have been on this journey with our loved ones through dementias and Alzheimer's Disease, we have experienced and learned a lot that we can pay forward to others who are on the journey or who will be on the journey.

Write a blog and share your lessons (blogs can be therapeutic, as well, if you're a writer). Volunteer to lead a dementias or Alzheimer's Disease support group, either online or in person. Volunteer at adult day care centers or assisted living facilities with memory care units. Offer to talk about it in the community and at church. Find ways to help other people with what you've learned and experienced.

Turn all of this into something that can help others and you will find that there is a great deal of healing and peace that comes from that. You will also find that paying it forward makes it all worth it.

Although none of us would have wanted for our loved ones to go through these neurological diseases, because they did and invited us along for the duration, their suffering left a legacy to us that they would want us to share with the future.

I pray for the best for each of you who reads these words not just now, but in the future. Take good care, my friends.

Song List for Book Title and Chapter Titles

Book Title: "You Oughta Know" – Alanis Morissette

Chapter 1: "I Don't Remember" – Peter Gabriel

Chapter 2: "Brain Damage" – Pink Floyd

Chapter 3: "Disconnection Notice" – Sonic Youth

Chapter 4: "White Rabbit" – Jefferson Airplane

Chapter 5: "Clocks" – Cold Play

Chapter 6: "Starry, Starry Night" – Don Mclean

Chapter 7: "Purple Haze" – Jimi Hendrix

Chapter 8: "Can't Find My Way Home" - Traffic

Chapter 9: "Fallin'" – Alicia Keys

Chapter 10: "Walk It Back" – R. E. M.

Chapter 11: "Unwell" – Matchbox 20

Chapter 12: "The Dignity Song" – Frank Horvat (music) & Adam Nihmey (lyrics)

Chapter 13: "Teach Your Children" – Crosby, Stills, Nash & Young

Chapter 14: "Old and Wise" – Alan Parsons Project

Chapter 15: "A World Unseen" – Rosanne Cash

www.ingramcontent.com/pod-product-compliance
Lightning Source LLC
Chambersburg PA
CBHW060508290526
45791CB00001B/318